Marijuana

DRUGS OF ABUSE
A Comprehensive Series for Clinicians

Volume 1   MARIJUANA
             Mark S. Gold. M.D.

Marijuana

Mark S. Gold, M.D.

Fair Oaks Hospital
Summit, New Jersey

Plenum Medical Book Company
New York and London

Library of Congress Cataloging in Publication Data

Gold, Mark S.
  Marijuana.
  (Drugs of abuse; v. 1)
  Includes bibliographies and index.
  1. Marijuana. I. Title. II. Series. [DNLM: 1. Cannabis. 2. Cannabis Abuse. 3. Cannabinoids—pharmacology. WM 276 G618m]
RC568.C2G64   1989   616.86'3   88-32427
ISBN 0-306-43062-2

© 1989 Plenum Publishing Corporation
233 Spring Street, New York, N.Y. 10013

Plenum Medical Book Company is an imprint of Plenum Publishing Corporation

Printed in the United States of America

Preface

Marijuana is the most widely used illicit drug in America. Some 40% of the adult population has tried marijuana at least once. It is the third largest agricultural commodity in the nation and a $10 billion industry. In many areas of the country, marijuana production or sale is the largest moneymaker by far. In Florida, for example, it ranks ahead of every business except tourism.

It is also a widely misunderstood substance. An entire generation of Americans grew up believing that marijuana was virtually risk-free. This belief persists, despite growing evidence of physical, psychological, and social harm that is caused by the drug.

The worst victims of this misinformation are young people. They, of all groups, are the least equipped to uncover and objectively evaluate the evidence regarding marijuana. At the same time, they are the most at risk for long-term problems resulting from marijuana use.

v

As physicians we must make every effort to guide young
people away from this drug.

There are very significant dangers in young people
experimenting with marijuana. The drug detoxification
center at our hospital—and centers throughout the
country—are packed with middle-class young people
who started out smoking pot. None of them intended
to become addicted, but the fact is that young people
are more vulnerable to the influence of the drugs and
become dependent easily. They may escalate usage, and
progress to use of other drugs.

Teenagers need to understand that addiction and
dependence are not matters of willpower, but are,
rather, functions of body chemistry and psychological
needs that are beyond individual will. Addiction occurs
to people in all walks of life, including highly accom-
plished businesspersons, physicians, and even religious
leaders. Many of them started out taking drugs to deal
with painful medical conditions or to cope with stresses
of professional life. A young person who has not yet
developed a strong personality and character can be extremely susceptible.

Studies also indicate that a large percentage of auto
accidents now involve alcohol and/or marijuana use, resulting in countless, needless deaths. Especially in the
suburbs, partying with drugs almost always involves
driving.

Young people should be asked; Is it worth getting
high if it means that one, two, or three of your friends
are going to forfeit their lives to addiction or to die in
accidents as a result? Put this way, many decide that it
is not. But for others the threat of death or addiction is
not a deterrent, and may actually encourage drug use.

Apart from tragic outcomes, adolescence happens to be the worst time, from a developmental standpoint, to engage in drug use. Physiologically, pot smoking may suppress the sex hormones, interfering with growth processes, sexual maturation, and menstruation. Any departures from the normal in this area may be acutely disturbing at an age when a person needs every reassurance of being physically normal. Long-term effects in this area of function are impotence, loss of normal sexual drive, and infertility.

Psychologically, adolescence is a time to develop self-awareness and a healthy sense of identity. A child who deals with personal uncertainties by "zonking out" to a drug-induced grandiosity is avoiding the necessary process of developing a firm sense of self. If anxieties about intimacy or confronting others are avoided by using drugs, the teenager postpones the task of learning how to become comfortable with others. Achievement of a sound identity will remain unresolved, which may be a factor in the prolonged "adolescence" that is so commonly seen—with individuals in their late twenties still wondering who they are and what they would like to do with their lives. Only by confronting fear-inducing situations can the fear be mastered and self-confidence nourished.

Using marijuana for performance anxieties related to schoolwork, or achievement in general, has similarly long-range repercussions. Students in our treatment programs sometimes boast that they get high several nights a week, even before exams, and still earn B grades. I answer that they are denying themselves the chance to learn how considerable their potential may be. Even to the A students, I point out how much more they might fulfill themselves and contribute to society if part of their brains were not incapacitated. Few of them realize, moreover, that the components of marijuana are stored in fatty tissue, including the brain, for weeks after ingestion, influencing and possibly impairing cognitive skills. I also suggest to these teenagers that, although they may be holding their own in school despite smoking pot, a stressful time may come in college or graduate school, when academic demands are much greater than those they are now experiencing. The danger lies in having already learned a "solution"— drugs—that the student under stress may then resort to.

Anyone faced with counseling teenagers about drug use may expect some clever rationalizations. For example, teenagers protest that adults can't understand how pot lets them see things "as they really are," and how it enhances interpersonal communication. They should be told that studies indicate just the opposite— that marijuana impairs perception and effective communication. One study, for example, involved pot-smoking and nonintoxicated subjects engaging in conversations. The stoned persons thought that the pairs were understanding one another profoundly—but they were generally unable to remember the thread of their own conversations and uttered non sequiturs that had nothing to do with their companions' statements. As for the argument "You don't understand," I point out that you don't have to have cancer to be an oncologist—or even the best oncologist. Similarly, you don't have to use drugs to understand drug abuse—in fact, it's better if you don't.

Young people might also be asked to evaluate honestly just how enjoyable or frightening the experience of being high is. Often it is more negative than enjoyable. The intoxicated person may feel terror about forbidden or self-destructive impulses. Paranoid states are common; best friends appear sinister, and every passing siren is believed to be the police coming to arrest the person who is high. It is only afterwards, in the company of their friends, that they reinterpret the experience as a "great time."

Young people questioned about the wisdom of smoking pot are quick to point out that their parents drink, and that pot is "no worse" than liquor. In the first place, the statistics on alcohol abuse and alcohol-related traffice fatalities show that alcohol is far from benign itself. In the second place, the known physical and psychological effects of marijuana indicate that it is indeed worse than alcohol.

Unfortunately, too many parents are taken in by this type of false logic, and reason that if it's okay for them to have a drink, they can't come down too hard on their children for smoking marijuana. In doing so, they abdicate their responsibilities as parents. Teenagers are not known for their moderation, and the children will almost certainly try to outdo their parents. If parents are heavy drinkers themselves, they must consider the consequences that these actions have for the future of their children, and reduce their own alcohol (or eliminate marijuana) consumption as an example to their children.

Young people are in the process of graduating from indulgence and fantasy fulfillment of childhood and learning to deal with the real world to gain their ends. They must learn that a sense of well-being comes from within themselves, from work, and from genuine relationships rather than from drug-fostered illusions. That is the specific developmental task of adolescence jeopardized by marijuana and other drugs.

I would like to thank Herbert Kleber, M.D., George Aghajanian, M.D., Boris Astrachan, M.D., and D. Eugene Redmond, M.D., of Yale University for encouraging me to pursue a career in substance abuse research. I would also like to thank Buddy Gleaton, Ed.D., Carlton Turner, Ph.D., Lee Dogoloff and Donald Ian MacDonald, M.D., for their outstanding work in the study of marijuana and its effects. Their important work has helped me apply my knowledge of cocaine and opiates to the field of marijuana research.

Mark S. Gold, M.D.

Summit, New Jersey

Contents

1

Marijuana Use and Abuse
An Overview

The risks and consequences of marijuana use have been intensively debated in the United States for more than 50 years. Unfortunately, the discussion has often relied more on rhetoric and hysteria than on objective scientific evidence. More than simply a medical issue, the controversy over marijuana has been defined in terms of beliefs, values, and political persuasion.

However valid these various perspectives may be, they have created a troubling climate for physicians. In an effort to lend scientific support for their positions, proponents and opponents alike have selectively cited or dismissed the scientific research that has been conducted, and have drawn conclusions that go far beyond the limits justified by the underlying evidence. Anecdotal evidence has been presented as conclusive and poorly controlled or even discredited studies continue to be referenced. Perhaps most disturbing is the practice of citing the *lack* of evidence as evidence itself—that is, of citing inconclusive studies as evidence of marijuana's safety.

Although much of this confusion has been generated by advocates who lack rigorous scientific training, it has muddied the waters for physicians who require a clear and objective understanding of the risks of marijuana abuse. In addition, it has clouded the physician's role. The physician's concern with marijuana use is very straightforward: Does it cause health problems? If so, how can these problems be prevented or treated?

The answer to the first is an unequivocal yes. Marijuana use has been shown to cause a variety of physical and psychological problems. Although some of these disorders are still the subject of scientific debate, many of them are well established. Moreover, they are progressive rather than self-limiting, and are responsive to medical treatment. Thus, the justification for medical intervention is clear.

An Overview of Cannabinoids

Cannabis sativa is an annual plant that grows both wild and under cultivation throughout the tropical and temperate zones. It may grow as high as 20 feet. (Formerly the Indian variety of marijuana was classified as a separate species—*C. indica*—but it has since been reclassified as a subspecies of *C. sativa*.)

Closely related to the hops plant (although very different in appearance), cannabis is dioecious—that is, it grows as separate male and female plants. The male plant is taller and usually dies after the flowering cycle.

The female, by contrast, is smaller and bushier. It secretes a resin that covers the flowering tops and nearby leaves. The resin is more abundant when the plant is grown in tropical areas, leading to speculation that its function is to retard moisture loss.

Traditionally, the flowering tops and adjacent leaves of the female have been cultivated for their psychoactive properties. Hashish consists primarily of the resin. It was long believed that male plants were not psychoactive; however, recent studies reveal that the males and females have similar potencies.[2]

The most common psychoactive compound in marijuana is delta-9-tetrahydrocannabinol (delta-9-THC), but the plant contains more than 60 related compounds known as cannabinoids.[1,3] Most of them have no known psychoactive properties and unknown physiological effects. Marijuana's psychoactive effects are predominantly caused by delta-9-THC.

The potency of marijuana varies greatly. When marijuana is grown by traditional methods, the highest concentration of cannabinoids is found in the flowers of the female plant. However, *sinsemilla*, a seedless version, has been widely cultivated by domestic growers in recent years, and concentrations of THC are much higher throughout the plant.

This increased potency has drastically changed the picture of marijuana use. For example, a typical marijuana cigarette in the early 1970s might contain 1% THC by weight and perhaps 10 mg of THC.[4] Today a high-quality marijuana cigarette might contain as much as 150 mg of THC—or twice as much if it is laced with hashish oil.[4] Thus the user today can easily be exposed to doses as high as 300 mg from a single joint. Studies have shown that a daily dose of 180 mg of THC a day for 11 to 21 days produces a defined withdrawal syndrome.[5]

Forms and Types of Marijuana

Marijuana and its derivatives are used in a variety of forms (Table 1) and go by a variety of names throughout the world, including "pot," "grass," "herb," "tea," "reefer," "mary jane," "ganja," "bhang," "charas," "kif," and "dagga." Marijuana is most often dried and smoked. It may be rolled into a cigarette (known as a joint, reefer, or, less commonly, spliff), or smoked in a pipe. Water pipes (sometimes called bongs or hookahs) are often used to humidify the smoke and permit deeper inhalation.

TABLE 1. Forms and Types of Marijuana

Marijuana
  Prepared from dried leaves and flowers of the *cannabis sativa* plant. Potency: 1% THC and up (early 1970s); 6–14% THC (current strains of domestic sinsemilla)
Hashish
  Prepared by collecting the resin secreted by cannabis leaves or by boiling the plant. It is pressed into bricks or cakes. Potency: 10–20% THC.
Hashish oil
  Prepared by distilling the plant in organic solvents. Potency: 15–30% THC.

SOURCES: Nahas GG: *Marijuana in Science and Medicine*. New York, Raven, 1984. Cohen S: Marijuana, in *American Psychiatric Association: Annual Review*. Washington, DC, American Psychiatric Press, vol 5, 1986. Mann P: *Marijuana Alert*. New York, McGraw-Hill, 1985. Gold MS: *The Facts About Drugs and Alcohol*. New York, Bantam, 1986.

Marijuana may be refined into hashish or the more potent hashish oil, which is then smoked. Any of these substances may also be ingested orally—typically baked into brownies or cookies—causing less potent but more long-lasting effects. THC is very insoluble in water, making it difficult to prepare injectable solutions—indeed, virtually the only known cases of intravenous administration of cannabinoids occur in research studies; the practice is virtually unknown among regular users.

The History of Marijuana Use

Cannabis sativa grows wild throughout most of the tropical parts of the world. Historically its seeds have been used for animal feed, its fiber for hemp rope, and its oil as a vehicle for paint. But its widest use throughout history has been for its intoxicating properties.

With alcohol and opium, marijuana is one of the oldest known intoxicants. The reason is simplicity itself: It requires only minimal cultivation and preparation before use.

The oldest known written record of marijuana* use comes from the records of the Chinese Emperor Shen Nung in 2727 B.C.[7] It is believed to have first been cultivated in Asia and was used in India as early as 2000 B.C. in religious ceremonies.[8,9] Written evidence of its use in the Middle East dates from about 500 A.D., though some have suggested that it is referred to in the Old Testament.[10,11] The ancient Greeks and Romans were

---

* The term *marijuana* (i.e., "Mary Jane") apparently comes from Mexico, where it was originally a slang term for cheap tobacco.[6]

familiar with cannabis; the Greek physicians Dioscordes and Galen mention it in connection with the treatment of otitis media, and Herodotus describes its being thrown upon hot stones to release its vapor.[12,13]

From the Middle East, the use of Cannabis spread throughout the Islamic Empire throughout North Africa. Its use was not without its detractors. The Emir Soudouni Schekhounia of Arabia outlawed it in 1378, and the Arab historian Al Magrii blamed the decline of Egyptian society on it.[14,15]

Cannabis spread to the western hemisphere in 1545, when Spaniards imported it to Chile for the use of its fiber.[16] It may have come by way of African slaves even earlier.[16] By the eighteenth century it was known in Europe. Carolus Linnaeus assigned it the name *Cannabis sativa* in 1735.[17]

Hemp was grown in the American settlements of Jamestown, Virginia, in 1611 and in New England by 1629. Though it was primarily grown during the colonial period for the manufacture of rope, but there is evidence that its psychoactive properties were known to the colonists. George Washington, for example, is known to have grown hemp at Mount Vernon, and careful study of his diaries have led some to conclude that he separated the potent female plants for his personal "medicinal" use.

Though the drug had been touted as a natural herbal cure and used by physicians in India, England, and Egypt, it was not used widely in the United States until the 1840s, when it became popularized within and outside of medical circles by the writings of Dr. W. B. Oshavghwessy, Jacques Joseph Moreau, and Fitz Hugh Ludlow.[8,18] From 1850 to 1942, cannabis was listed in the *U.S. Pharmacopeia,* and pharmaceutical firms such as Parke-Davis, Lilly, Squibb, and Burroughs-Wellcome marketed preparations containing cannabis.[7] "Hashish houses" emerged in large American cities during the last half of the nineteenth century, but use of the drug was limited to a small, fashionable group.[7] Marijuana use proliferated in the United States during the 1920s, perhaps partially as a result of soldiers' exposure to it in Central America and the Caribbean or due to Prohibition.

In 1937, marijuana was effectively outlawed by the federal Marijuana Tax Act. Its passage was due in large part to a campaign of hysteria and misinformation orchestrated by Harry J. Anslinger, the Commissioner of the Federal Bureau of Narcotics. Anslinger's portrayal of marijuana as a drug that immediately and irrevocably led to homicidal insanity did much to set the tone for very harsh criminal sanctions against the drug—including, in Georgia, the penalties of life imprisonment or death for selling marijuana to a minor.[7]

Marijuana use became widely popular within the youthful counterculture in the 1960s. Its use increased steadily through the 1960s and 1970s, peaking in 1979. Since then its use has declined dramatically.

Current-Use Patterns

When the use of marijuana first became widespread, most of the supplies came from foreign sources. Marijuana came primarily from South and Central America (bearing such names as Colombian Gold, Panama Red, and Acapulco Gold) or from the Orient (e.g.,

Thai sticks). Hashish and hash oil usually came from the Middle East or Mediterranean, often by way of Europe. Most of it entered the country through Florida and California, as well as major ports such as New York.

Although these foreign sources still exist, the marijuana scene has changed drastically in the past decade as a result of illicit domestic production. Faced with the need to grow marijuana clandestinely in relatively small areas, domestic producers have used sophisticated breeding and cultivation techniques to vastly increase the potency of their crop—and thus its market value. Indeed, marijuana is available on the street today that is hundreds of times more potent than the typical street pot of the late 1960s and early 1970s. This single fact has made obsolete much of what we once knew about the risks and consequences of marijuana use.

Who Uses Marijuana?

Two national surveys provide the best evidence available about who uses marijuana. The first, the National Household Survey, has been conducted regularly since 1971. It is based on a random sample of persons 12 years of age and older living in households in the coterminous United States. The Second, *Student Drug Use in America*, has sampled high school students since 1975; survey respondents include each year's high school students as well as a portion of the previous year's respondents. The surveys do not include certain groups: the first fails to reach those who do not have regular addresses or who live in institutional settings, such as military barracks or student dormitories; the second omits those who do not reach their senior year in high school. In light of evidence that both of these groups may be more likely to use marijuana, these studies probably understate marijuana use to some extent. Also, of course, they rely on self-reporting of illicit behavior, further suggesting that they understate actual use.

Even so, the results of these studies are illuminating (Table 2). Petersen[19] summarizes them as follows:

- Both marijuana experimentation and current use (within the month preceding the survey) have increased markedly since the 1960s. Between 1971 and 1982 [the latest year for which data was complete at the time of Petersen's report], the percentage of youth (ages 12 to 17) who had ever used [marijuana] nearly doubled—from 14% to 27.3%. Among those aged 18 to 25, an increase of over 50% occurred in the same period—from 39.3 to 64.3%. The percentage of those currently using (i.e., those reporting use in the 30 days prior to the survey) is roughly half that of those who have ever used. This has been a consistent pattern over time for young adults and adolescents.
- Among high school seniors, nearly half (47.3%) of the class of 1975 had experimented with marijuana, compared with about 60% of the classes of 1978 to 1982 and 50% in the class of 1987. As with other adolescent and young adult groups, the percentage of current users is approximately half that of those who have ever tried the drug.
- Daily use has not been surveyed in the National Household Survey, but among high school sen-

TABLE 2. High School Senior Drug Use: 1975–1986

	'75	'76	'77	'78	'79	Class of '80	'81	'82	'83	'84	'85	'86
						Ever used						
Marijuana/hashish	47%	53%	56%	59%	60%	60%	60%	59%	57%	55%	54%	51%
Inhalants[a]	NA	NA	NA	NA	18	17	17	18	18	18	18	20
Amyl & butyl nitrites	NA	NA	NA	NA	11	11	10	10	8	8	8	9
Hallucinogens[b]	NA	NA	NA	NA	18	16	15	14	14	12	12	12
LSD	11	11	10	10	10	9	10	10	9	8	8	7
PCP	NA	NA	NA	NA	13	10	8	6	6	6	5	5
Cocaine	9	10	11	13	15	16	17	16	16	16	17	17
Heroin	2	2	2	2	1	1	1	1	1	1	1	1
Other opiates	9	10	10	10	10	10	10	10	9	10	10	9
Stimulants[c]	NA	NA	NA	NA	NA	NA	NA	28	27	26	26	23
Sedatives	18	18	17	16	15	15	16	15	14	13	12	10
Barbiturates	17	16	16	14	12	11	11	10	10	10	9	8
Methaqualone	8	8	9	8	8	10	11	11	10	8	7	5
Tranquilizers	17	17	18	17	16	15	15	14	13	12	12	11
Alcohol	90	92	93	93	93	93	93	93	93	93	92	91
Cigarettes	74	75	76	75	74	71	71	70	71	70	69	68

Used in last year

Marijuana/hashish	40%	45%	48%	50%	51%	49%	46%	44%	42%	40%	41%	39%
Inhalants[a]	NA	NA	NA	NA	8	6	6	7	6	7	8	9
Amyl & butyl nitrites	NA	NA	NA	NA	6	6	4	4	4	4	4	5
Hallucinogens[b]	NA	NA	NA	NA	7	11	10	9	8	7	8	8
LSD	7	6	6	6	7	7	7	6	5	5	4	5
PCP	NA	NA	NA	NA	7	4	3	2	3	2	3	2
Cocaine	6	6	7	9	12	12	12	12	11	12	13	13
Heroin	1	1	1	1	1	1	1	1	1	1	1	1
Other opiates	6	6	6	6	6	6	6	5	5	5	6	5
Stimulants[c]	NA	NA	NA	NA	NA	NA	NA	20	18	18	16	13
Sedatives	12	11	11	10	10	10	11	9	8	7	6	5
Barbiturates	11	10	9	8	8	7	7	6	5	5	5	4
Methaqualone	5	5	5	5	6	7	8	7	5	4	3	2
Tranquilizers	11	10	11	10	10	9	8	7	7	6	6	6
Alcohol	85	86	87	88	88	88	87	87	87	86	86	85
Cigarettes	NA	NA	NA	NA	NA	NA	NA	NA	NA	NA	NA	NA

Used in past month

Marijuana/hashish	27%	32%	36%	37%	37%	34%	32%	29%	27%	26%	26%	23%
Inhalants[a]	NA	NA	NA	NA	3	3	3	3	3	3	3	3
Amyl & butyl nitrites	NA	NA	NA	NA	2	2	1	1	1	1	2	1

(cont.)

TABLE 2. (cont.)

	Class of											
	'75	'76	'77	'78	'79	'80	'81	'82	'83	'84	'85	'86
Hallucinogens[b]	NA	NA	NA	NA	5	4	5	4	4	3	4	4
LSD	2	2	2	2	2	2	3	2	2	2	2	2
PCP	NA	NA	NA	NA	2	1	1	1	1	1	2	1
Cocaine	2	2	3	4	6	5	6	5	5	6	7	6
Heroin	*	*	*	*	*	*	*	*	*	*	*	*
Other opiates	2	2	3	2	2	2	2	2	2	2	2	2
Stimulants[c]	NA	NA	NA	NA	NA	NA	NA	11	9	8	7	6
Sedatives	5	5	5	4	4	5	5	3	3	2	2	2
Barbiturates	5	4	4	3	3	3	3	2	2	2	2	2
Methaqualone	2	2	2	2	2	3	3	2	2	1	1	1
Tranquilizers	4	4	5	3	4	3	3	2	3	2	2	2
Alcohol	68	68	71	72	72	72	71	70	69	67	66	65
Cigarettes	37	39	38	37	34	31	29	30	30	29	30	30
	Daily users											
Marijuana/hashish	6.0%	8.0%	9.1%	10.7%	10.3%	9.1%	7.0%	6.3%	5.5%	5.0%	4.9%	4.0%
Inhalants[a]	NA	NA	NA	NA	0.1	0.2	0.2	0.2	0.2	0.2	0.4	0.4
Amyl & butyl nitrites	NA	NA	NA	NA	0.0	0.1	0.1	0.0	0.2	0.1	0.3	0.5

LSD	0.0	0.0	0.0	0.0	0.0	0.0	0.1	0.0	0.1	0.1	0.1	0.0
PCP	NA	NA	NA	NA	0.1	0.1	0.1	0.1	0.1	0.1	0.3	0.2
Cocaine	0.1	0.1	0.1	0.1	0.2	0.2	0.3	0.2	0.2	0.2	0.4	0.4
Heroin	0.1	0.0	0.0	0.0	0.0	0.0	0.0	0.0	0.1	0.0	0.0	0.0
Other opiates	0.1	0.1	0.2	0.1	0.0	0.1	0.1	0.1	0.1	0.1	0.1	0.1
Stimulants[c]	NA	NA	NA	NA	NA	NA	NA	0.7	0.8	0.6	0.4	0.3
Sedatives	0.3	0.2	0.2	0.2	0.1	0.1	0.2	0.2	0.2	0.1	0.1	0.1
Barbiturates	0.1	0.1	0.2	0.1	0.0	0.1	0.1	0.1	0.1	0.0	0.1	0.1
Methaqualone	0.0	0.0	0.0	0.0	0.0	0.1	0.1	0.1	0.0	0.0	0.0	0.0
Tranquilizers	0.1	0.2	0.3	0.1	0.1	0.1	0.1	0.1	0.1	0.1	0.0	0.0
Alcohol	5.7	5.6	6.1	5.7	6.9	6.0	6.0	5.7	5.5	4.8	5.0	4.8
Cigarettes	26.9	28.8	28.8	27.5	25.4	21.3	20.3	21.1	21.2	18.7	19.5	18.7

[a] Inhalants—adjusted for underreporting of amyl and butyl nitrites.
[b] Hallucinogens—adjusted for underreporting of PCP.
[c] Stimulants—adjusted for overreporting of nonprescription stimulants.
NA indicates data not available
* Indicates less than 0.5%

Terms

Ever used: Used at least one time.
Used in last year: Used at least once in the 12 months prior to survey.
Used in past month: Used at least once in the 30 days prior to survey.
Daily users: Used 20 or more times in the month before survey.
SOURCE: National Institute on Drug Abuse, Monitoring the Future Study, 1986

iors, it rose from 6 to nearly 11% between 1975 and 1978 and has since fallen to 3.3% in the class of 1987.

Petersen noted other significant findings from the National Household Survey and other studies. Briefly, these studies showed that:

- The lower the age of initial use of alcohol and cigarettes, the more likely the individual is to use marijuana
- The age of first use of marijuana has decreased steadily
- Daily use of marijuana (i.e., 20 or more days per month) is positively correlated with absenteeism and poor academic performance and negatively correlated with religious involvement and plans to attend college
- Daily use is more common among seniors who are socially active and who spend little time at home
- Use of other drugs is much more common among seniors who use marijuana on a daily basis than among less frequent users; nearly half of daily marijuana users currently use amphetamines and almost a third of them use cocaine.

The National Household Surveys show that marijuana is the most popular illicit drug used in the United States.[20] A recent national survey indicated that some 15 million Americans smoke marijuana at least monthly; 9 million smoke it at least once a week; and 6 million smoke it daily.[21] In 1987, 1 high school senior in 25 smoked marijuana every day; nearly 1 in 4 are current users.[22,23] Half of high school seniors report that they have tried the drug (Table 2). More than half of all marijuana users report that they first tried the drug between the sixth and ninth grades.[24] Males are more likely to be users than females.[19]

Marijuana is often used in conjunction with other drugs. The 1984 senior survey showed that 5% of daily marijuana users also reported daily alcohol use; 7% reported current (i.e., in the preceding 30 days) use of amphetamine or cocaine, and 2% current use of other illicit drugs.[25] Recent reports indicate a new form of marijuana known as AMP that is soaked in formaldehyde.[26] Other adulterants that have been reported include insect spray, LSD, amphetamines, strychnine, stramonium leaves, rat poison, and catnip.[27,28] The herbicide paraquat has been found on marijuana samples in the past as a result of government eradication programs in Mexico, but the practice has been discontinued. Adulterants may cause acute psychosis and physical toxicity.

Marijuana use is not only widespread but evenly distributed. In the early 1960s its use was largely confined to urban coastal areas, but currently its use is fairly uniform across regions and in both urban and rural communities.

Surveys show that marijuana use by high school seniors increased steadily from the late 1960s to 1979, at which time it began to drop.[29] Many rationales have been offered to explain the recent decline, including the development of effective prevention and educational programs and a generalized swing to more conservative values among students.

Although the figures showing a decline in use are

encouraging, two new trends are not so reassuring. First, the initiation into marijuana use is beginning at earlier and earlier ages. The second trend is the vastly increased potency mentioned previously. Little is known about the developmental effects of marijuana when its use begins in childhood or very early adolescence; in addition, the long-term effects of high-potency strains of marijuana have never been studied, because these strains never existed until just a few years ago. Each of these trends alone is alarming enough; together they present some very troubling—and still unanswered—questions.

Indeed, they even cast some doubt on the validity of the trend seen in the survey data referred to above. As pointed out in *Marijuana and Health*, the 1982 Institute of Medicine study, the decline could simply be an artifact, with heavy users of marijuana becoming increasingly underrepresented in the survey sample (i.e., high school seniors) due to absenteeism and dropouts associated with earlier and more intensive involvement with the drug.[29]

Affected Ages

The 1985 National Household Survey revealed that 62 million Americans—roughly a third of the population older than 12—have tried marijuana at least once. Among persons aged 18 to 25, some 5 million (about 60%) have done so.[30] The same source showed that 19.9% of youths (ages 12 to 17), 36.8% of young adults (ages 18 to 25) and 9.5% of older adults (26 years of age and older) used marijuana in the preceding year. Current users (i.e., use within the preceding 30 days) among these same groups were, respectively 12.2%, 22%, and 6.5%, respectively.[21] With the exception of the 26+ group, these figures have shown a considerable decline from their peaks in 1979. For example, current use among these groups in 1979 versus 1985 was 16.7 versus 12.2%; 35 versus 22%; and 6 versus 6.5%, respectively. The figures for lifetime use and use within the preceding 30 days show similar trends.

Use during the 18-to-25 age span seems to be mostly due to social factors rather than to underlying psychological problems and in many cases, cessation of use occurs spontaneously once the user reaches early adulthood. In fact, those cases where onset of use occurs before age 13 or after age 24 are far more likely to involve psychiatric disorders, and these persons are at very high risk of progressing to addiction.[21]

Correlates of Marijuana Use

Marijuana use has been correlated with poor academic performance, low academic motivation, delinquent behavior, problems with authority, and lack of self-esteem.[19] However, studies show that in most cases these psychosocial problems *preceded* initiation into marijuana use. It is not known whether marijuana use *per se* exacerbates these tendencies, but it is clearly part of a complex picture of psychosocial dysfunction.

There is evidence that the acceptability of marijuana among adolescents is on the decline: whereas only 35% of the high school seniors in 1978 considered regular use a "great risk," 58% of them felt that it was by 1981.[31] The Student Drug Use Survey showed that current use

TABLE 3. Trends in Perceived Harmfulness of Drugs (Percentage Saying "Great Risk")[a]

Q. How much do you think people risk harming themselves (physically or in other ways), if they . . .	Year of graduation													'86–'87 change
	1975	1976	1977	1978	1979	1980	1981	1982	1983	1984	1985	1986	1987	
Try marijuana once or twice	15.1	11.4	9.5	8.1	9.4	10.0	13.0	11.5	12.7	14.7	14.8	15.1	18.4	+3.3ss[b]
Smoke marijuana occasionally	18.1	15.0	13.4	12.4	13.5	14.7	19.1	18.3	20.6	22.6	24.5	25.0	30.4	+5.4sss
Smoke marijuana regularly	43.3	38.6	36.4	34.9	42.0	50.4	57.6	60.4	62.8	66.9	70.4	71.3	73.5	+2.2
Try LSD once or twice	49.4	45.7	43.2	42.7	41.6	43.9	45.5	44.9	44.7	45.4	43.5	42.0	44.9	+2.9
Take LSD regularly	81.4	80.8	79.1	81.1	82.4	83.0	83.5	83.5	83.2	83.8	82.9	82.6	83.8	+1.2
Try PCP once or twice	NA	NA	NA	NA	NA	NA	NA	NA	NA	NA	NA	NA	55.6	NA
Try cocaine once or twice	42.6	39.1	35.6	33.2	31.5	31.3	32.1	32.8	33.0	35.7	34.0	33.5	47.9	+14.4sss
Take cocaine occasionally	NA	NA	NA	NA	NA	NA	NA	NA	NA	NA	NA	54.2	66.8	+12.6sss
Take cocaine regularly	73.1	72.3	68.2	68.2	69.5	69.2	71.2	73.0	74.3	78.8	79.0	82.2	88.5	+6.3sss
Try heroin once or twice	60.1	58.9	55.8	52.9	50.4	52.1	52.9	51.1	50.8	49.8	47.3	45.8	53.6	+7.8sss
Take heroin occasionally	75.6	75.6	71.9	71.4	70.9	70.9	72.2	69.8	71.8	70.7	69.8	68.2	74.6	+6.4sss
Take heroin regularly	87.2	88.6	86.1	86.6	87.5	86.2	87.5	86.0	86.1	87.2	86.0	87.1	88.7	+1.6

Try amphetamines once or twice	35.4	33.4	30.8	29.9	29.7	29.7	26.4	25.3	24.7	25.4	25.2	25.1	29.1	+4.0ss
Take amphetamines regularly	69.0	67.3	66.6	67.1	69.9	69.1	66.1	64.7	64.8	67.1	67.2	67.3	69.4	+2.1
Try barbiturates once or twice	34.8	32.5	31.2	31.3	30.7	30.9	28.4	27.5	27.0	27.4	26.1	25.4	30.9	+5.5sss
Take barbiturates regularly	69.1	67.7	68.6	68.4	71.6	72.2	69.9	67.6	67.7	68.5	68.3	67.2	69.4	+2.2
Try one or two drinks of an alcoholic beverage (beer, wine, liquor)	5.3	4.8	4.1	3.4	4.1	3.8	4.6	3.5	4.2	4.6	5.0	4.6	6.2	+1.6s
Take one or two drinks nearly every day	21.5	21.2	18.5	19.6	22.6	20.3	21.6	21.6	21.6	23.0	24.4	25.1	26.2	+1.1
Take four or five drinks nearly every day	63.5	61.0	62.9	63.1	66.2	65.7	64.5	65.5	66.8	68.4	69.8	66.5	69.7	+3.2s
Have five or more drinks once or twice each weekend	37.8	37.0	34.7	34.5	34.9	35.9	36.3	36.0	38.6	41.7	43.0	39.1	41.9	+2.8
Smoke one or more packs of cigarettes per day	51.3	56.4	58.4	59.0	63.0	63.7	63.3	60.5	61.2	63.8	66.5	66.0	68.6	+2.6
Approximate N =	(2804)	(2918)	(3052)	(3770)	(3250)	(3234)	(3604)	(3557)	(3305)	(3262)	(3250)	(3020)	(3315)	

[a] Answer alternatives were: (1) No risk, (2) Slight risk, (3) Moderate risk, (4) Great risk, and (5) Can't say, drug unfamiliar.

[b] Level of significance of difference between the two most recent classes: s = .05, ss = .01, sss = .001.

SOURCE: 1987 High School Senior Survey.

of illicit drugs dropped from 39 percent in 1978 and 1979 to 29 percent in 1984.[32]

Recent studies show that high school students increasingly perceive marijuana as a dangerous drug—a trend that reflects that seen for other drugs as well. (See Table 3) In 1987, 73.5% of seniors felt that people who smoke marijuana regularly are at "great risk"—up from a low of 34.9% in 1979. This stunning reversal parallels the diminished use of marijuana among seniors, and it suggests that the drop in use is not an artifact, but rather reflects a real change in attitudes toward marijuana and drugs in general. At the same time, it powerfully suggests that education about risks *does* have a major and beneficial impact on use patterns.

Controversies

Many of the controversies over marijuana use and research into marijuana-related health problems are discussed in the chapters that follow. There are several, however, that are of such a broad nature that they are best addressed individually.

Limitations of Scientific Evidence

Despite the long history of marijuana use, careful scientific research of its effects did not begin until the early 1970s. Several types of studies have been employed, but all have limitations. Epidemiological evidence of health problems—such as that linking cigarette smoking with heart disease and lung cancer—requires years of use by large populations. Even then, it may not be clear whether observed effects are due to the substance or to other concurrent factors. With marijuana, epidemiologic studies are further complicated by its illegality (which affects the accuracy of reports of its use), changes in the drug itself (with potency increasing vastly over the past decade) and changing patterns of use (with use becoming more and more prevalent among adolescents and children).

Laboratory studies, on the other hand, seldom reflect the realities of actual use. For ethical, practical, and legal reasons, the duration of use is limited—usually to no more than a few weeks. Because of the variability in marijuana, researchers typically use laboratory extracts of THC, administered by a variety of routes, or government-grown marijuana of established potency and purity. In actual practice, however, the user's supplies may vary widely in potency, and may have any number of adulterants or impurities. In addition, they may use marijuana in conjunction with other drugs, with unknown interactions.

In an attempt to assess the long-term effects of marijuana, some researchers have studied cultures wherein its use is traditional. These studies, too, have severe limitations. In other cultures, marijuana's use may be socially sanctioned, often within a religious or ceremonial context. These social norms tend to establish certain clear limits for marijuana use. In the United States, by contrast, marijuana use is part of an illicit drug culture, and its use is often an expression of rebelliousness or rejection of mainstream values. In this context, it is plausible to conclude that there is a greater likelihood of abuse (as the limiting social norms are absent), and introduction to other drugs that are common within this drug culture.

Furthermore, the physical effects are likely to differ as well. In cultures where marijuana use is traditional, it is commonly mixed with tobacco, which probably causes users to inhale less deeply and exhale more quickly than those who smoke marijuana alone. Although the significance of these differences are unknown, the differing health effects of smoking cigarettes versus smoking pipes or cigars suggest that smoking styles may be very important.[33] Finally, the impact of additional confounding variables makes any extrapolation to a modern industrial society tentative at best. Endemic infectious diseases, poor diet, inadequate public-health measures, and an emphasis on physical labor rather than intellectual achievement in day-to-day life are just some of the realities of Third World cultures that make it difficult to correlate clinical observations with the use or nonuse of marijuana or to relate these findings to our own culture.

Is Marijuana Safe?

Much of the controversy concerning marijuana since the late 1960s has involved its risks. Marijuana advocates consistently characterize it as a safe drug—in the words of one, "[Smoking a joint is] as OK as having a glass of wine with dinner or champagne to celebrate an event."[34] At the opposite end of the spectrum is the government-sponsored hysteria of the 1930s, which portrayed marijuana use as leading inevitably and immediately to homicidal insanity. Obviously the truth lies somewhere in between.

A dispassionate assessment of the known health effects of marijuana permits a rough comparison of its risks to other substances. For example, the risk of lung cancer among regular chronic users is roughly comparable to that of tobacco cigarettes. Motor impairment is similar to that seen with alcohol, but it lasts far longer. It is clearly a major factor in automobile accidents and other instances of trauma. Thus, at the very least marijuana has physical risks that probably exceed those of alcohol and cigarettes *combined*. In light of the fact that tobacco and alcohol use are widely recognized as two of the most significant public health problems in the United States, and the fact that marijuana use is widespread, this evidence alone is sufficient to classify marijuana use as a major public-health problem.

But research reveals that marijuana entails other risks as well. It is a major risk factor for the development of substance-abuse problems involving cocaine, narcotics, and other illicit drugs. And recent evidence shows that new powerful strains of marijuana now on the market have major addictive potential. Finally, there are well-established adverse effects on the immune and reproductive systems, the cardiovascular and pulmonary systems, and on psychosocial functioning and development. In light of all this evidence—as well as the sobering thought that our ignorance of this drug far exceeds our knowledge—it can only be concluded that marijuana is far from the benign substance that many of its users believe it to be.

The Gateway Concept

One significant controversy is whether marijuana use causes the use of other illicit drugs such as heroin

TABLE 4. Cocaine Use among
Adults Aged 18 and Over by
Lifetime Frequency of
Marijuana Use

Frequency of marijuana use	Ever used cocaine (%)
Never	0.3
1–2 times	6.0
3–5 times	10.4
6–10 times	18.8
11–49 times	32.3
50–99 times	50.3
100–199 times	58.9
200 + times	77.3

SOURCE: 1985 National Household Survey on Drug Abuse

or cocaine. It is clear that marijuana use often progresses to use of additional illicit drugs, and the use of such drugs is almost *always* preceded by marijuana use (see Table 4).[35–40] What is subject to debate is whether the relationship is causative or simply correlative.

Logic and evidence support the idea that this relationship is causative. Much of the controversy over the issue of causation stems from a semantic confusion. The epidemiological definition of causation is based on the following criteria[41]:

- The two variables in question (e.g., marijuana use and use of other illicit drugs) are statistically associated
- The presumed causative variable (in this case,

marijuana use) is temporally prior to the other variable
- The association between the two variables remains even after the effects of other variables that are prior to both of them are removed
- The association has not been demonstrated to be spurious

This definition differs in subtle ways from the classic experimental demonstration of causation, but it would be impossible to design a strict double-blind study to answer the question of whether marijuana use causes the use of other illicit drugs.* Both approaches have their strengths and weaknesses. For example, in an epidemiological study, marijuana users are self-selected. And although case-matched studies can control for known or suspected variables, there may be other unknown confounding variables. With a classic double-blind study the issue is not validity but relevance: the constraints imposed by the design do not necessarily reflect typical real-life experiences.

Ultimately, the question is one of utility. It is clear

---

* Incidentally, the same issues exist with regard to the link between cigarettes and lung cancer. Pro-tobacco advocates argue that the epidemiological link between the two is correlational rather than causative—in other words, that underlying or intervening factors are involved. In the absence of any credible evidence of such factors, such an argument must be regarded as specious.

Interestingly, the epidemiologic link between marijuana use and subsequent use of other illicit drugs is much stronger than that between cigarettes and cancer.[42] Those who argue against a causative interpretation suggest underlying social or psychological disorders that lead to both. Careful study has thus far failed to identify any such disorder.

that the epidemiological evidence has very important implications for prevention. They show that, in the real world, marijuana use is a *necessary precursor* to the use of such drugs as heroin and cocaine. In this context the issue of causation becomes largely irrelevant; what is important is that those who use marijuana are at significant risk for progression to other drugs, and thus are appropriate candidates for intervention. The ultimate significance of the "gateway drug" concept is that marijuana use is an important signal of the need for intervention.

Although the question of causation is irrelevant to the need for intervention, it does shed light on the nature that these interventions should take. Case histories and clinical experience universally point to social factors as the mechanism of causation: Marijuana use introduces the user to a social milieu in which other drugs are more accepted and more readily available. Thus, preventive and treatment efforts must be aimed not only at physical abstinence, but at altering the psychosocial and behavioral patterns (such as peer-group identification) that accompany it.

The Legalization Issue

Should marijuana be legalized? It should not. However, from a strictly scientific perspective, the question can be framed more narrowly: Do legal sanctions against marijuana prevent or reduce the incidence of marijuana use? In short, do these laws have their intended effect?

Recent history offers some guidance on this question. Proponents of legalization draw an analogy with the failure of Prohibition. They point out that Prohibi-

tion failed to stop people from drinking; it simply drove
the liquor industry into the hands of organized crime
and deprived the nation of tax revenues. The repeal of
Prohibition gave the government the ability to regulate
alcohol more effectively, and prevented fruitless efforts
to enforce an unenforceable law. For similar reasons,
they argue, marijuana should be legalized and regulated
to ensure quality, limit access to those of legal age, and
to disrupt the link between marijuana smoking and
other illicit activities.

This analogy has a number of flaws, however. The
most important is that whereas Prohibition attempted
to change a status quo in which alcohol consumption
was already well-established, legalization of marijuana
would change the status quo in a way that promotes
acceptance of marijuana use. Legalizing marijuana gives
the appearance of a governmental "seal of approval" for
a practice that now has considerable social stigma, at
least in the mainstream culture. Despite any disclaimers
to the contrary, it seems virtually certain that legalization would reinforce the view that marijuana is relatively
benign—a view that is at odds with the scientific
evidence.

When considering the legalization question, a more
relevant example than Prohibition is the change in public perception about cigarette smoking that has occurred
in the 1970s and 1980s. Although cigarettes have not
been outlawed, extensive legal restrictions have been
imposed on smokers and the tobacco industry. Unlike
Prohibition, these restrictions have been implemented
with broad public support. Why?

There seem to be two major reasons. First, Prohibition was an issue couched in *moral* terms—alcohol was

seen as "sinful" by those who attempted to restrict its use. Whether one agreed with this position or not was simply a matter of opinion. Restrictions on cigarettes, by contrast, are justified on the basis of public health rather than morality. And despite the efforts of the tobacco companies to challenge the scientific evidence, there is no real disagreement about the fact that cigarette smoking is harmful. Closely related to this is the fact that the public has been exposed to a massive, long-term educational campaign about the hazards of cigarettes. Significantly, facts rather than hysteria have turned the tide of public opinion.

There is some evidence that the facts about marijuana are proving to be similarly effective. In addition to the declining-use patterns among adolescents are the results of a survey in which increasing numbers of high school students say they believe that marijuana is very dangerous.[31]

It is likely that some of the shift in public attitudes—even among those who once used marijuana and other illicit drugs—has come from publicity over the cocaine epidemic. During the late 1960s and 1970s, cocaine was widely touted as a safe and nonaddictive drug. As the facts about cocaine emerged, they caused many current and former users to question the notion of "safe" recreational drugs. Events of recent years have reinforced the old pharmacologic truism that all drugs carry risks.

References

1. Turner CE: Cannabis: The plant, its drugs, and their effects. *Aviation Space Environ Med* 1983;54:363–368.

2. Pillard RC: Marihuana. *N Engl J Med* 1970;283:294.
3. Turner CE: *The Marijuana Controversy: Definition of Research Perspectives and Therapeutic Claims.* American Council for Drug Education, 1981.
4. Mann P: *Marijuana Alert.* New York, McGraw-Hill, 1985.
5. Jones RT, Benowitz W, Bachman I: Clinical studies of cannabis tolerance and dependencies. *Ann NY Acad Sci* 1976;282:21–239.
6. Snyder BH: *Uses of Marijuana.* New York, Oxford University Press, 1971.
7. Brecher EM et al: *Licit and Illicit Drugs: The Consumers Union Report on Narcotics, Stimulants, Depressants, Inhalants, Hallucinogens, and Marijuana—Including Caffeine, Nicotine and Alcohol.* Boston, Little, Brown, 1972.
8. Nahas GG: *Keep Off the Grass.* New York, Pergamon, 1979.
9. Nahas GG: *Marijuana in Science and Medicine.* New York, Raven, 1984.
10. Creighton C: On Indications of the Hashish-vice in the Old Testament. *Janus* 1902;8.
11. Clay M: *The Song of Solomon in the Book of Grass.* New York, Grove, 1967.
12. Walton RP: *Marijuana: America's New Drug Problem.* Philadelphia, Lippincott, 1938.
13. Giannini AJ, Slaby AE, Giannini JD: *Handbook of overdoses and detoxification emergencies.* New York, Medical Examination Publishing, 3rd ed, 1985.
14. Rosenthal F: *The Herb Hashish versus Moslem Medieval Society.* Leiden, Netherlands, E. J. Brill, 1972.
15. Lewin L: *Phantastica: Narcotic and Stimulating Drugs—Their Use and Abuse.* [Reprint of 1924 edition.] New York, Dutton, 1964.
16. Hoffman F: *A Handbook on Drug and Alcohol Abuse.* Oxford University Press, 2nd ed, 1983.
17. Winek CL: Some historical aspects of marijuana. *Clin Toxicol* 1977;10:243–253.
18. Grinspoon L, Bakalar JB: Marihuana. In Lowinson JH, Ruiz P, eds: *Substance Abuse: Clinical Problems and Perspectives.* New York, Williams and Wilkins, 1981.
19. Petersen RD: Marijuana overview, in Glantz MD: *Correlates and Consequences of Marijuana Use.* Rockville, MD, National Institute on Drug Abuse, 1984.

20. Fishburne PM, Abelson HI, Cisin I: *National Survey on Drug Abuse: Main Findings: 1979*. Washington, DC: U.S. Government Printing Office, 1980 [DHHS publication no. (ADM) 80–976].
21. National Institute of Drug Abuse: *NIDA Capsules: Highlights of the 1985 National Household Survey on Drug Abuse*. Rockville, MD, 1986.
22. National Institute of Drug Abuse: *NIDA Capsules: High School Senior Drug Use 1975–1986*. Rockville, MD, 1987.
23. Schwartz RH: Marijuana: An overview. *Ped Clin North Am* 1987;34(2):305–317.
24. Anonymous: Alcohol and other drug abuse among adolescents. *Metropolitan Insurance Company Statistical Bulletin* 1984;65(7):4–73.
25. Kandel D: Adolescent drug abuse. *J Am Acad Child Psych* 1982;20:573–577.
26. Millman RB, Sbriglio R: Patterns of use and psychopathology in chronic marijuana users. *Psych Clin North Am* 1986;9(3):533–545.
27. Yamaguchi K, Kandel DB: Patterns of drug use from adolescence to young adulthood. II. Sequence of progression. *Am J Public Health* 1984;74:668–672.
28. Jessor R, Jessor SL: *Problem behavior and psychosocial development: a longitudinal study of youth*. New York, Academic, 1977.
29. Institute of Medicine: *Marijuana and Health*. Washington, DC, National Academy, 1982.
30. Miller JA, Cisin IH: Highlights from the National Survey on Drug Abuse 1979. Washington, DC, U.S. Government Printing Office, 1980 [DHHS publication no. (ADM) 80-1302].
31. Johnston LD, Bachman JG, O'Malley PM: Highlights from Student Drug Use in America, 1975–1981. NIDA, Washington, DC, U.S. Government Printing Office, 1981. [DHHS publication no. (ADM)82-1208.]
32. Johnston LD, O'Malley PM, Bachman JA: *Use of licit and illicit drugs by America's high school students: National trends* 1975–1984. Washington, DC, U.S. Government Printing Office, 1985. [DHHS publication no. (ADM) 85-1394].
33. Petersen RC: Importance of inhalation patterns in determining effects of marijuana use. *Lancet* 1979:727–728.
34. O'Driscoll P: Marijuana users still test the law. *USA Today* 1987; Jul 30:A1–A2.

35. MacDonald DI: Patterns of alcohol and drug abuse among adolescents. *Pediatr Clin North Am* 1987;34(2):275–288.
36. Kanor DB, Logan JA: Patterns of drug use from adolescence to young adulthood: I. Periods of risk for initiation, continued use, and discontinuation. *Am J Public Health* 1984;74:660–666.
37. Johnston LD, O'Malley PM, Bachman JG: *Use of licit and illicit drugs by America's high school students: 1975–1984.* Rockville, MD, National Institute on Drug Abuse, 1985.
38. Yamaguchi K, Kandel DB: Patterns of drug use from adolescence to young adulthood: III. Predictors of progression. *Am J Public Health* 1984;74:673–81.
39. Yamaguchi K, Kandel DB: Patterns of drug use from adolescence to young adulthood. II. Sequence of progression. *Am J Public Health* 1984;74:673–681.
40. Gold MS: Users ever younger: Pot is "gateway" drug for adolescents. *Alcoholism and Addiction* 1986;6(4):14.
41. O'Donnell JA, Clayton RR: The steppingstone hypothesis: a reappraisal [abstract], in Glantz MD: *Correlates and consequences of marijuana use.* Rockville, MD, National Institute on Drug Abuse, 1984.

2

Cannabinoid Pharmacology

Marijuana is a unique psychoactive agent; its chemistry and pharmacology do not fit well within any other class of mind-altering drugs. In low doses it has paradoxical effects, acting both as a stimulant and depressant. In higher doses depressant effects predominate.[1] In addition to its action on the central nervous system (CNS), marijuana also affects the immune system, reproductive system, and cardiovascular system.[1]

Though marijuana is widely used, its pharmacology is poorly understood. It is often difficult to draw firm conclusions from the research that has been conducted, for a number of reasons. First, marijuana is not a single drug, but a complex mix: More than 60 cannabinoid compounds have been isolated from marijuana smoke. Further, measurements of active levels of cannabinoids in body tissues is difficult because of their high potency; doses as low as 10 μg of delta-9-THC per kg of body

37

weight are sufficient to cause a "high."[2] In addition, marijuana's effects vary widely across species, and long-term effects are difficult to extrapolate from short-term human studies.

These and other methodological complexities help explain why uncertain and often contradictory results that have been obtained in marijuana research since the 1960s. For example, some researchers have conducted studies using "standard" marijuana cigarettes supplied by the federal government; others have used preparations of marijuana extracts—primarily delta-9-tetrahydrocannabinol (delta-9-THC). Dosages have varied widely in different studies, as have the mode of ingestion (oral, intravenous, inhalation) and vehicles (ethanol, Tween 80, DMSO, and others). In addition, the subjects in these studies are not easily comparable; for obvious reasons, many studies have been conducted in vitro or using animal subjects. Human subjects have at times included nonusers, "moderate" users, and "heavy" users—categories that are often inconsistent from one study to another.

The studies are also complicated by the increasing potency of illicit marijuana over the past two decades. With today's marijuana being, on the average, about five times as powerful as that of the 1960s, the current "moderate" user would be ingesting much larger doses of cannabinoids than the average "heavy" user of, for example, 1977. And, finally, virtually all of the experimental studies involving humans have looked at *short-term* effects; practical considerations make long-term or longitudinal studies all but impossible to conduct.

For all these reasons, current research offers only a very sketchy outline of the pharmacology and effects of marijuana. Despite the fact that it is one of the most widely abused psychoactive drugs in the world, we know far less about it than, for example, narcotics (whose effects and chemistry are relatively straightforward), or such synthetic compounds as amphetamines and benzodiazepines (which, because of their therapeutic value, have been studied under controlled conditions and in well-defined populations). These caveats must be kept in mind when considering the conclusions presented in this chapter.

Of the 60-odd cannabinoids found in marijuana smoke, only 14 have been studied in depth: delta-9-THC*—the most common and most psychoactive one; delta-8-THC; cannabidiol (CBD); and cannabinol (CBN). Behavioral studies in animals also show that various constituents found in marijuana have additive or antagonistic effects, a fact that helps explain the varying potencies found in different marijuana preparations— and the often inconsistent results of experimental studies.

Some debate has existed over whether marijuana's main constituent—delta-9-THC—acts directly on the CNS, or whether it first must be metabolized to 11-OH-delta-9-THC, which studies have shown to be more potent than the parent compound. However, recent studies—for example, one in which delta-9-THC was in-

---

* Two different numbering schemes exist for cannabinoids. The more common dibenzopyran system is used here. In addition, it must be kept in mind that a number of cannabinoid isomers exist. The (−)-*trans* isomer of delta-8-THC and delta-9-THC—which are the most pharmacologically active as well as the ones that occur naturally in the marijuana plant—are the ones referred to in this discussion.

jected directly into the cerebroventricle of squirrel monkeys—support the idea that delta-9-THC is directly psychoactive, and need not be converted metabolically to produce its effects.[3]

Pharmacokinetics

A key factor in the pharmacokinetics of cannabinoids—and one that distinguishes them from the majority of drugs—is that they are highly soluble in lipids, although showing only very slight solubility in water. This fact seems to play an important role in the way they are metabolized and in their psychoactive effects, although the mechanism of these actions is far from clear. In addition, cannabinoids' lipid solubility helps explain the extremely long half-life of these compounds, because they are retained by lipids within the body.

Route of Administration

Smoking. The most common route of administration of cannabinoids—at least when they are used illicitly—is by smoking. Marijuana smoke contains approximately 0.3% to >3% delta-9-THC (about 10% in hashish).[4] It also contains numerous other substances, including other cannabinoids (which may exert unknown synergistic or antagonistic effects) as well as tars, carbon monoxide, and most other substances found in tobacco smoke (with the exception of nicotine).

The actual amount of THC ingested by smoking depends on a number of factors: (1) the speed at which it is smoked, (2) puff duration, (3) volume inhaled, and

(4) the amount of time the user withholds expiration after inhalation.[2,4] The use of a pipe does significantly increase cannabinoid transfer: About 20% of delta-9-THC present in marijuana is transferred when a marijuana cigarette is smoked in its usual fashion, versus about 45% with a pipe.[5,6] Two factors that users widely believe to affect potency—humidification (by use of a water pipe) and the type of cigarette paper—do not influence the percentage of transfer of delta-9-THC.[7]

In addition to active smoking, persons may be passively exposed to marijuana smoke in social situations. Some controversy exists over whether such passive smoking can produce intoxication (a "contact high"). One study found that some subjects showed subjective and physiologic effects after passive exposure to extremely heavy exposure (16 marijuana cigarettes). Subjective effects were mild after passive exposure to the smoke of 4 marijuana cigarettes (and were not significantly different from placebo responses), but were more pronounced after exposure to the smoke of 16 marijuana cigarettes. *Physiologic* effects, by contrast, were mild and highly variable; in most cases, the difference in physiologic response between marijuana and placebo failed to reach significant levels, even after exposure to the smoke of 16 marijuana cigarettes.[8] Curiously, however, this same exposure resulted in urine cannabinoid levels similar to those seen after active smoking of one marijuana cigarette.

Ingestion. Orally ingested delta-9-THC is converted by intestinal acids into 11-hydroxy-delta-9-THC, a compound with a pharmacological profile virtually identical to delta-9-THC. Ingestion produces effects similar to those seen with smoking; however, they are less intense and of longer duration.

IV Administration. Generally, intravenous administration of cannabinoids has been limited to research studies, because of the limited availability of purified delta-9-THC and the difficulty of preparing IV solutions. In general, plasma profiles with IV administration are the same as for smoking.[9] However, some difficulties occur because of the insolubility of cannabinoids in water. Various vehicles have been used, such as Tween 80 and ethanol, but their use may affect study results—especially ethanol, whose psychoactive effects are similar in many respects to those of the cannabinoids.

Mechanism of Action

Surprisingly little is known about cannabinoids' mechanism of action. One study raises the possibility that cannabinoids may act on benzodiazepine receptors. In addition, cross-tolerance of cannabinoids with ethanol and other depressants raises the possibility that some of their effects are due to general CNS depression. Some researchers have suggested that they act on specific cannabis receptors. No such receptors have been identified, but as alterations to the THC structure erase the psychoactive effects, it seems plausible that a specific receptor is matched to psychoactive THCs.[10]

At least some of the differences among psychoactive THCs may be caused by differences in penetration, distribution, or elimination from the CNS.[11] This seems to be the case with delta-9-THC and 11-OH-delta-9-THC.[12–14] Although some drugs have been shown to reverse or block cannabis effects, Martin suggests that these phenomena are more likely due to drug interactions (i.e., indirect action) than to specific antagonism.[15]

The Compartment Model

The time relationship between cannabinoid administration and serum levels is complex; moreover, subjective psychological effects do not correlate well with serum levels. This fact suggests a complex mechanism of action, possibly involving a one- or two-compartment model. Chiang *et al.* describe an empirical two-compartment model to describe the lag, and note that one to four hours after smoking a marijuana cigarette, effects are directly proportional to mean THC levels.[16]

Effects of Cannabinoids

Effects of Chronic Use

One of the most unusual findings regarding delta-9-THC is that of Lemberger *et al.*, who concluded that it disappears more quickly from the plasma of chronic users than that of nonusers[17]; however, this finding has been challenged by others.[18] What is clear is that persons with a history of heavy use achieve higher plasma levels of delta-9-THC than naive users who smoke the same amount of marijuana; presumably the difference is due to more efficient smoking techniques.[19,20]

Behavioral Effects

The reported subjective psychological effects of cannabinoids—which include excitement and dissociation of ideas, enhancement of the senses, distortions of time and space, delusional thinking, impulsiveness, illusions, and hallucinations—are accompanied by objective behavioral changes, including a deterioration of psychomotor performance, diminished attention span and memory, and reduced physical strength.[1]

Animal studies of cannabinoids reveal widely varying behavioral effects, but several appear consistently. One is a hyperreflexive response to specific stimuli accompanying the overall sedative effects. This sedative/hyperreflexive effect results in unusual behavioral responses. For example, groups of white mice exhibit a so-called "popcorn" response: when one mouse lands on another mouse, it in turn jumps, causing a chain reaction that eventually subsides as all the mice become sedated once again.[21]

This sedative/hyperreflexive combination is unique among CNS depressants. Although some other depressants and stimulants may show paradoxical effects under certain circumstances, none of them do so with the consistency of cannabinoids, and only the cannabinoids cause hyperreflexia throughout the period of CNS depression.[21]

Animals receiving delta-9-THC sleep a great deal in the 24 hours following administration[22]; when aroused, they exhibit hyperreflexive behavior. These and other effects show that cannabinoids have a very long duration of action—24 hours or more, and an even longer half-life (see the following section).

Effects on Motor Skills

Marijuana clearly causes a deterioration of motor skills. For example, 94% of those whose plasma concentrations of delta-9-THC exceeded 25–30 ng/ml failed a standard roadside sobriety test administered ninety minutes after smoking—despite the fact that by plasma levels of THC had dropped drastically by the time the test was administered. Some 60% of them failed the test one hundred fifty minutes after smoking.[23]

The effects on motor skills has particular relevance to the role of marijuana in traffic accidents and other types of accidents. Although epidemiological studies are hampered by methodological difficulties—in particular, the poor correlation between blood levels of cannabinoids and their effects—experimental studies show that marijuana impairs many of the fundamental skills needed for safe driving, including coordination, tracking, perception, and vigilance. Similarly, performance in driving simulators and on the road is demonstrably poorer after marijuana use.[24] Studies further demonstrate that the impairment of marijuana and alcohol on driving skills are additive.[24]

These results are generally consistent with findings that the marijuana "high" persists long after plasma THC levels have dropped. Thus, unlike alcohol, delta-9-THC plasma levels alone are a poor indicator of marijuana-related motor skill impairment. In general, motor skills are impaired for hours or even days after use.

One study of pilots who were exposed to marijuana found significant impairment in flying skills as long as 24 hours after impairment. Especially disturbing is the fact that the pilots themselves were unaware of their impairment.[25]

These effects on motor skills have significant implications regarding the consequences of marijuana use. Especially the fact that these effects persist for relatively long periods of time after use—and that this carry-over effect is not perceived by the user nor accurately reflected in blood-THC levels—suggests that the role of marijuana in traffic accidents and other types of accidents is vastly underestimated. Indeed, marijuana arguably poses a greater risk to drivers even than alcohol, whose effects are relatively short-lived and accompanied by a subjective sense of intoxication.

Assessment of the risks of drugs tends to focus on *direct* effects, but these and similar studies demonstrate that the *indirect* effects may be even more profound. Although it is difficult to estimate these effects with accuracy, they must be considered as part of the overall cost—to the individual and to society—of drug abuse.

Effects on Cognitive Functioning

The effect of marijuana on attention has been studied using a variety of cognitive tests.[26] These studies show that subjects consistently do more poorly after receiving even moderate amounts of marijuana. Some of the specific impairments found have included confusion, loss of directedness, and the ability to simultaneously remember information (for example, numbers) and manipulate it to achieve a goal.

Other studies show that marijuana's effects on attention are marked but complex.[26] Short-term memory appears to be affected more strongly than does retrieval of information that is already present in memory. In word-recognition tests, where subjects are asked to identify words that were previously read aloud to them, subjects receiving marijuana tended to accept more incorrect words from a list that was supplied to them, and when asked to write as many words as they could recall, were able to remember fewer words than subjects receiving placebo. In tests of free recall—in which subjects are given a book to read and later asked to recall the contents—those receiving marijuana recalled less and included fewer content words. Experimental evidence has not confirmed the perceived enhanced sensory awareness (e.g., visual or auditory acuity) reported by users.[26]

Amotivation and Aggression

An often-cited, but anecdotal, consequence of marijuana use is *amotivational syndrome*—a loosely defined concept involving disinterest, apathy, and antisocial behavior. Some of these effects are characteristic of CNS depressants in general. Whether a distinct amotivational syndrome can be ascribed to marijuana use is open to question. The term is imprecise, though it is clear from clinical observation that some adolescents who use marijuana appear flat in affect and devoid of the drive and energy normally seen in adolescents.

As a CNS depressant, marijuana would be expected to *decrease* aggression. However, animal studies generally show that delta-9-THC *increases* aggressive behavior—especially in animals who are deprived of food or sleep or otherwise stressed.[27,28] For example, administration of marijuana extract or delta-9-THC causes aggression in rats that have been deprived of food for twenty hours,[29–31] and increases deaths among rats.

Other studies, however, cloud this picture. Low doses (0.5 and 1 mg/kg) of delta-9-THC *reduced* schedule-induced aggression in pigeons,[32] whereas delta-8- and delta-9-THC reduced isolation-induced aggressiveness in mice and Chinese hamsters.[33] One group of researchers studying the effects of cannabinoids on sleep-deprived rats concluded that their effects depend on the animals' state, producing CNS depression in normal rats but increasing aggressiveness and irritability when administered to stressed rats.

We have no clear understanding of how cannabinoids affect the neurotransmitter system to cause or potentiate aggression in laboratory animals. Large doses of atropine-block cannabis-induced aggression in sleep-deprived rats, suggesting that the cholinergic nervous system is involved.[31] Other studies point to a role for dopamine and serotonin in cannaboid-induced aggression.[28,34]

For the most part, cannabinoids' effects on aggression are inconsistent across species, and Dewey's review of the literature concludes that these and other studies are *not* predictive of cannabinoids' effects on aggression in human beings.

Tolerance

The development of tolerance to the effects of cannabinoids is difficult to characterize. For example, one study failed to find significant tolerance to the effects of delta-9-THC—as measured both by pulse rate and subjective reports—unless subjects repeatedly self-administered large doses of the drug.[35] In another study, regular marijuana users reported increased elation after smoking marijuana, but their pulse rates showed no significant increase.[36] In the same study, intermittent and occasional smokers exhibited the opposite effects, with *no* significant marijuana-induced elation, but *did* show significant increases in pulse rate. In other words, regular use of marijuana seems to intensify (and thus presumably reinforce) the subjective "high." When these subjects were given oral nabilone (a synthetic cannabinoid) and oral delta-9-THC, they experienced a significant increase in pulse rate but no elation. These results are confusing and to some extent counterintuitive. However, one unequivocal finding from the study was that among these three compounds, marijuana proved to the most powerful reinforcer by far.

Some researchers have suggested that marijuana tolerance is *dispositional*—that is, caused by changes in the way the drug is stored or metabolized.[37] Others, including Agurell *et al.*, believe that tolerance is primarily functional, a conclusion supported by studies showing similar patterns of drug distribution and metabolism in heavy users and light users.

Correlation between Plasma Levels and Subjective Effects

Taken alone, plasma levels of psychoactive cannabinoids and subjective reports of the "high" are not closely correlated. However, when these two values are charted against time on a graph (see Figure 1), a revealing pattern emerges. After intravenous administration of delta-9-THC, plasma levels drop quickly at first, and then more slowly. The subjective "high," however,

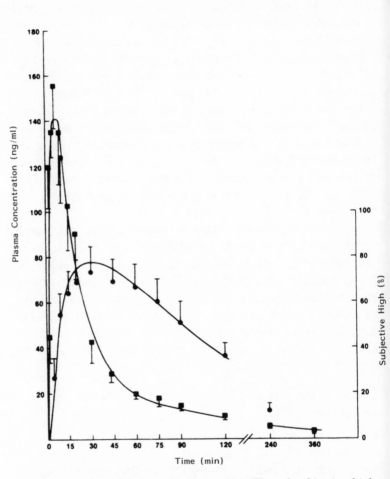

Figure 1. Plasma THC concentration-time (■) and subjective high-time (●) after smoking one 2.5% THC cigarette ($\bar{X} \pm$ SE; $n = 6$). *Solid curves* are computer fits to the data.

rises to a sharp peak over the first thirty minutes, and then drops off gradually and uniformly.

As noted previously, this pattern has led some to speculate that delta-9-THC must first be metabolized to 11-hydroxy-delta-9-THC before it becomes psychoactive.[38] According to this theory, the initial drop in delta-9-THC levels represents conversion to 11-hydroxy-delta-9-THC, which in turn accounts for the rise in the subjective "high." However, if this theory were correct, IV administration of 11-hydroxy-delta-9-THC would be expected to create an instantaneous "high." It does not; in fact, it shows a pattern virtually identical to that of delta-9-THC.[39,40]

Another possible explanation—though not well supported by experimental studies—is that the lag observed on the graph is caused by slow penetration of psychoactive cannabinoids into the brain.[41] Agurell et al.[37] suggest that the reasons could involve "the time required to start the biochemical effects or, speculatively, to penetrate to the receptor, or displace a possible endogenous ligand"; however, they caution that these explanations are only speculation, and that causes of the lag remain unknown.[33]

Formation and Excretion of Metabolites

Some 80 metabolites of delta-9-THC are known.[42] Of these, 7-hydroxy-delta-9-THC and 6[beta]-hydroxy-delta-9-THC are capable of producing marijuana-like symptoms and increased pulse rate. The others are believed to be essentially nonpsychoactive. About two-thirds of these metabolites are excreted in feces and about one-third in the urine. As noted previously, the metabolites are excreted slowly, with only about half the dose eliminated after two to three days.[42] In fact, traces of cannabinoid metabolites may be found as long as several weeks after marijuana.[18] Neither delta-9-THC nor CBD are excreted unchanged in the urine, although traces of CBN may be found. Delta-9-THC is excreted in feces.[42]

Anticonvulsant Effects of Cannabinoids

At least one cannabinoid—cannabidol (CBD)—shows some anticonvulsant action, and researchers have investigated its potential as a anticonvulsant medication. Because it is chemically unrelated to other anticonvulsants, it could offer an alternative for those in whom other drug therapies fail to control seizures. Studies of CBD's anticonvulsant properties have been rare, in large part because of the difficulty of preparing CBD, and thus far inconclusive.[43,44]

Summary

As the preceding discussion shows, some facets of cannabinoid pharmacology are understood with a fair degree of certainty, whereas for others the evidence is inconclusive and contradictory. In general, the psychoactive components of marijuana exert an overall depressive effect on the central nervous system, with some paradoxical stimulatory components. They are very potent, with active plasma levels in the nanogram range, but even in relatively high doses they do not possess the immediately life-threatening potential of such other psychoactive drugs as opiates, cocaine, barbiturates, or alcohol.

Cannabinoids are soluble in lipids, but almost entirely insoluble in water. It is likely that they are bound up in fatty tissues, and slowly excreted from these tissues over the course of several days, accounting for their long half-life.

The psychoactive mechanism(s) of these drugs are unknown, although the bulk of current evidence suggests that they act on some type of receptors. Though chemically unrelated to other psychoactive compounds, the evidence suggests that may act to some degree on similar sites within the CNS. For example, they show some cross-tolerance with ethanol, and appear to exert antianxiety and anticonvulsant effects via benzodiazepine receptors. A few cannabinoids show antiemetic activity.

Beyond this handful of relative certainties, however, many controversies continue to surround the pharmacology of cannabinoids. For example, their long-term effects—over the course of years, versus the days or weeks that typical studies examine—are controversial but largely unexplored for our culture. The reasons for these gaps are numerous. Certainly the drugs' illicit nature, as well as the almost total lack of a therapeutic role for them, make long-term studies difficult. Another less obvious, but still important, factor is marijuana's low-acute toxicity; unlike the case with heroin or cocaine, acute marijuana use, in and of itself, rarely comes to the attention of emergency physicians. But though marijuana's effects are far less dramatic than those of "killer drugs'' such as heroin or cocaine, it does not follow that it is harmless. As discussed in the chapters that follow, marijuana is definitely contraindicated for those in whom the developmental process is not yet complete— that is, children and adolescents. Unfortunately, this is the very group that uses it most heavily.

Because patients will often deny the consequences of long-term marijuana use—for obvious reasons—it is exceedingly difficult to establish links between illness and long-term use through population studies. For example, adolescents commonly enter emergency rooms with problems that they attribute to cocaine overdose or problems, even though they have been using marijuana before or simultaneously with the cocaine. Similarly, auto accidents are often attributed to alcohol use despite the fact of concurrent marijuana use. For all these reasons, the true incidence of marijuana-induced effects are unknown, and almost certainly understated.

References

1. Dewey WL: Cannabinoid pharmacology. *Pharmacol Rev* 1986;38(2):151–178.
2. Agurell S, Halldin M, Lindgren JE, et al: Pharmacokinetics and metabolism of delta-1-tetrahydrocannabinol and other cannabinoids with emphasis on man. *Pharmacol Rev* 1986;38(1):23.
3. Lemberger L, McMahon R, Archer R: The role of metabolic conversion on the mechanisms of actions of cannabinoids. In Braude MC, Szara S, eds: *Pharmacology of Marihuana*. New York, Raven, 1976, vol 1, 125–133.
4. Agurell S, Halldin M, Lindgren JE, et al: Pharmacokinetics and metabolism of delta-1-tetrahydrocannabinol and other cannabinoids with emphasis on man. *Pharmacol Rev* 1986;38(1):22.
5. Agurell S, Leander K: Stability, transfer, and absorption of can-

nabinoid constituents of cannabis (hashish) during smoking. *Acta Pharm Suec* 1971;8:391–402.

6. Davis KH Jr, McDaniel IA Jr, Cadwell LW, Moody PL: Some smoking characteristics of marijuana cigarettes, in Agurell S, Dewey WL, Willette RE (eds): *The Cannabinoids: Chemical, Pharmacologic, and Therapeutic Aspects.* New York, Academic, 1984:97–109.

7. Perez-Reyes M, Diguiseppi S, Davis KH, Schindler VH, Cook CE: Comparison of effects of marijuana cigarettes of three different potencies. *Clin Pharmacol Ther* 1982;31:617–624.

8. Cone EJ, Johnson RE: Contact highs and urinary cannabinoid excretion after passive exposure to marijuana smoke. *Clin Pharmacol Ther* 1986;40:247–256.

9. Agurell S, Halldin M, Lindgren JE, et al: Pharmacokinetics and metabolism of delta-1-tetrahydrocannabinol and other cannabinoids with emphasis on man. *Pharmacol Rev* 1986;38(1):40.

10. Harvey DJ: Pharmacology, metabolism, pharmacokinetics, and analysis of the cannabinoids, in *ISI Atlas of Science: Pharmacology 1987.* Philadelphia, ISI, 1987:209–210.

11. Martin BR: Cellular effects of cannabinoids. *Pharmacol Rev* 1986;38(1):54.

12. Schou J, Prockop LD, Dahlstrom G, Rohde C: Penetration of delta-9-tetrahydrocannabinol and 11-OH-delta-9-tetrahydrocannabinol through the blood-brain barrier. *Acta Pharmacol Toxicol* 1977;41:33–38.

13. Perez-Reyes M, Simmons J, Brine D, Kimmel GL, Davis KH, Wall ME: Rate of penetration of delta-9-tetrahydrocannabinol and 11-hydroxy-delta-9-tetrahydrocannabinol to the brain of mice, in Nahas G (ed): *Marihuana: Chemistry, Biochemistry, and Cellular Effects.* New York, Springer-Verlag, 1976:179–185.

14. Gough AL, Olley JE: Catalepsy induced by intrastriatal injections of delta-9-THC and 11-OH-delta-9-THC in the rat. *Neuropharmacology* 1978;17:137–144.

15. Martin BR: Cellular effects of cannabinoids. *Pharmacol Rev* 1986;38(1):56.

16. Chiang CWN, Barnett G, Brine D: Systemic absorption of delta-9-tetrahydrocannabinol after ophthalmic administration in the rabbit. *J Pharm Sci* 1983;72:136–138.

17. Lemberger L, Silberstein SD, Axelrod J, Kopin IJ: Marihuana:

Studies on the disposition and metabolism of delta-9-tetrahy-drocannabinol in man. *Science* 1970;170:1320–1322.

18. Dackis CA, Pottash ALC, Annitto W, Gold MS: Persistence of urinary marijuana levels after supervised abstinence. *Am J Psychiatry* 1982;139:1196–1198.

19. Ohlsson A, Lindgren JE, Wahlen A, Agurell S, Hollister LE, Gillespie HK: Plasma delta-9-tetrahydrocannabinol concentrations and clinical effects after oral and intravenous administration and smoking. *Clin Pharmacol Ther* 1980;28:409–416.

20. Ohlsson A, Lindgren JE, Wahlen A, Agurell S, Hollister LE, Gillespie HK: Single dose kinetics of deuterium labelled delta-1-tetrahydrocannabinol in heavy and light cannabis users. *Biomed Mass Spectrom* 1982;9:6–10.

21. Dewey WL: Cannabinoid pharmacology. *Pharmacol Rev* 1986;38(2):153.

22. Dewey WL: Cannabinoid pharmacology. *Pharmacol Rev* 1986;38(2):154.

23. Reeve VC, Grant JD, Robertson W, Gillespie HK, Hollister LE: Plasma concentrations of delta-9-tetrahydrocannabinol and impaired motor function. *Drug and Alcohol Dependence* 1983;11:167–175.

24. Moskowitz H: Marihuana and driving. *Accid Anal & Prev* 1985;17:323–345.

25. Yesavage J, Leirer VO, Ditman J, Hollister LE: "Hangover" effects of marijuana intoxication on aircraft pilot performance. *Am J Psychiatry* 1985;142:1325–1329.

26. Murray JB: Marijuana's effects on human cognitive functions, psychomotor functions, and personality. *J Gen Psychol* 1986;113(1):23–55.

27. Fujiwara M, Ibii N, Kataoka Y, Ueki S: Effects of psychotropic drugs on delta-9-tetrahydrocannabinol-induced long-lasting muricide. *Psychopharmacology* 1980;68:7–13.

28. Carlini EA, Lindsey CJ: Effect of serotonergic drugs on the aggressiveness induced by delta-9-tetrahydrocannibinol in REM-sleep-derived rats. *Braz J Med Biol Res* 1982;15:281–283.

29. Fujiwara M, Ueki S: The course of aggressive behavior induced by a single injection of delta-9-tetrahydrocannabinol and its characteristics. *Physiol Behav* 1979;22:535–539.

30. Carlini EA, Hamaoui A, Martz RMW: Factors influencing the

aggressiveness induced by delta-9-tetrahydrocannabinol in food-deprived rats. *Br J Pharmacol* 1972;44:794–804.

31. Musty RE, Lindsey CJ, Carlini EA: 6-Hydroxydopamine and the aggressive behavior induced by marihuana in REM sleep-deprived rats. *Psychopharmacology* 1976;48:175–179.

32. Cherek DR, Thompson T, Kelly T: Chronic delta-9-tetrahydrocannabinol administration and schedule-induced aggression. *Pharmacol Biochem Behav* 1980;12:305–309.

33. Ten Ham M, Van Noordwijk J: Lack of tolerance to the effects of two tetrahydrocannabinols on aggressiveness. *Psychopharmacology* 1973;29:171–176.

34. DeSouza, Neto JP: Effects of anti-acetylcholine drugs on aggressive behavior induced by cannabis sativa in REM sleep-deprived rats. *J Pharm Pharmacol* 1978;30:591–2.

35. Babor TF, Mendelson JH, Greenberg I, Kuehnle JC: Marihuana consumption and tolerance to physiological and subjective effects. *Arch Gen Psych* 1975;32:1548–1552.

36. Mendelson JH, Mello NK: Reinforcing properties of oral delta-9-tetrahydrocannabinol, smoked marijuana, and nabilone: Influence of previous marijuana use. *Psychopharmacology* 1984;83:351–356.

37. Agurell S, Halldin M, Lindgren JE, et al: Pharmacokinetics and metabolism of delta-1-tetrahydrocannabinol and other cannabinoids with emphasis on man. *Pharmacol Rev* 1986;38(1):28.

38. Lemberger L, Weiss JL, Watanabe AM, Galanter IM, Wyatt RJ, Cardon PV: Delta-9-tetrahydrocannabinol: Temporal correlation of the psychological effects and blood levels after various routes of administration. *N Engl J Med* 1972;286:685–688.

39. Lemberger L, Crabtree RE, Rowe HM: 11-Hydroxy-delta-9-tetrahydrocannabinol: Pharmacology, disposition, and metabolism of a major metabolite of marihuana in man. *Science* 1972;170:1320–1322.

40. Perez-Reyes M, Timmons MC, Lipton M, Davis KH, Wall ME. Intravenous injection in man of delta-9-tetrahydrocannabinol and 11-hydroxy-delta-9-tetrahydrocannabinol. *Science* 1972;177:633–635.

41. Agurell S, Halldin M, Lindgren JE, et al: Pharmacokinetics and metabolism of delta-1-tetrahydrocannabinol and other cannabinoids with emphasis on man. *Pharmacol Rev* 1986;38(1):31.

42. Agurell S, Halldin M, Lindgren JE, et al: Pharmacokinetics and metabolism of delta-1-tetrahydrocannabinol and other cannabinoids with emphasis on man. *Pharmacol Rev* 1986;38(1):34.
43. Ames FR, Cridland S: Anticonvulsant effect of cannabidiol, letter. *S Afr Med J* 1986;69:14.
44. Cunha JM, Carlini EA, Pereira AE et al: Chronic administration of cannabidiol to healthy volunteers and epileptic patients. *Pharmacology* 1980;21:175–185.

3

Medical Problems Associated with Marijuana Use

Marijuana* causes a number of medical problems, including respiratory ailments, impaired immunity, and reproductive disturbances. Often the symptoms are subtle and nonspecific, and the link with marijuana use not immediately apparent; thus, a careful history is important. Although acute respiratory discomfort can be eased with symptomatic treatment, abstinence is the only effective long-term treatment for all of these conditions. The limited evidence from long-term studies suggests that most of the medical effects are reversible with cessation of marijuana use. However, the psychological and developmental effects of marijuana on ad-

* Except where specifically noted, the term *marijuana* in this chapter refers to marijuana and its derivatives, including hashish, hashish oil, and delta-9-tetrahydrocannabinol (delta-9-THC).

olescents—as with other developmental injuries—may not be reversible.

A special concern is marijuana use during pregnancy. Numerous studies show that maternal marijuana use has direct deleterious effects on the developing fetus. A link between marijuana use and low birth weight is well-established; similarly, marijuana has been shown to increase the risk of complications during pregnancy. In addition, case reports and animal research strongly suggests that marijuana is a teratogen—a finding that is consistent with its known mutagenic and carcinogenic properties—and that it can cause fetal hypoxia resulting in impaired growth, prematurity, and fetal brain damage.

Respiratory Effects

Inhaled smoke from any source harms lung tissue and epithelial cells lining the airways, as well as the immune cells found in the lungs. All of these effects can make the lungs more vulnerable to infection, and can complicate or trigger respiratory disorders.[1]

Marijuana and tobacco smoke are chemically similar (except that marijuana smoke contains cannabinoids and tobacco smoke contains nicotine), and the effects of marijuana smoking parallel those seen in tobacco smokers. Smoking habits of the two groups are not identical; marijuana users tend to smoke less, but they inhale more deeply, do not use filters, and smoke the cigarette down to the butt. Thus, it seems reasonable to conclude that marijuana smoking carries similar risks of lung cancer, emphysema, chronic bronchitis, and other respiratory ailments as does cigarette smoking.

The cardiovascular effects of tobacco, however, are

related to nicotine. Although cannabinoids are known to cause short-term cardiovascular changes, these effects are very different from those caused by nicotine. The long-term consequences on the cardiovascular system are essentially unknown, and cannot be extrapolated from evidence related to cigarette smoking.

Acute Effects

The acute effects of marijuana smoking on ventilation are dose-dependent.[2] Smaller doses—one cigarette or less—stimulate ventilation, in conjunction with an increased metabolic rate and heightened response to CO_2 as a regulatory stimulant. Larger doses, by contrast, may have the opposite effect. Curiously, intravenous administration of delta-9-THC has relatively little effect on ventilation rates or respiratory response to CO_2.

Marijuana smoke is a powerful bronchodilator, persisting as long as sixty minutes after smoking. Again, delta-9-THC administered intravenously has much less potent bronchodilatory action, though its pulmonary effects may persist as long as six hours. The mechanism of action for bronchodilation is not clear, but involves neither beta-adrenergic stimulation nor blockade of receptors in smooth muscle.[3]

In addition to bronchodilation, heavy marijuana smoking (at least four days per week for six to eight weeks) results in mild airway obstruction.[4] One study found that these effects were incompletely reversed one week after cessation of smoking, suggesting that long-term heavy marijuana smoking "could lead to clinically significant and less readily reversible impairment of pulmonary function."[5]

Contaminated marijuana may result in respiratory infections or other disease. The use of paraquat herbicide on illegal marijuana crops is well-publicized. Marijuana harvested after it has been sprayed with paraquat can result in severe lung damage. Currently, the spraying of marijuana crops with paraquat has been discontinued by law enforcement authorities; however, its use in the future has not been precluded.[6]

In addition to chemical contamination, marijuana may also be contaminated by infectious agents, especially aspergillus organisms. One researcher found aspergillus in 11 of 12 marijuana samples tested.[7] Aspergillus can cause severe respiratory infections, as well as subacute infections that may easily be overlooked.[8]

Chronic Effects

Studies of hashish-smoking American soldiers stationed in West Germany have revealed a number of respiratory ailments associated with heavy hashish use. One study involved 31 soldiers who smoked 100 gm or more of hashish a month for 6 to 15 months. The study found that the primary ailments in this group were respiratory (bronchitis, sinusitis, asthma, and rhinopharyngitis).[9] A third of the soldiers had sputum-producing coughs, difficulty in breathing, and wheezing after 3 to 4 months of hashish use. Chest radiographs and sputum cultures were normal, and antibiotics failed to resolve the symptoms.

The condition—which was so severe that all of the affected soldiers were unable to work and four required hospitalization—resolved after they decreased their hashish consumption. Pulmonary tests administered three days after they reduced their intake of hashish showed mild airway obstruction. The patients responded to isoproterenol, leading the researchers to surmise that reversible bronchospasm, accumulation of fluid in the bronchi, or both, were responsible for the symptoms.

Another study of 200 soldiers who sought medical attention for problems related to hashish smoking found that inflammation of the mouth and back of the throat and persistent rhinitis were common.[10] Symptoms were relieved by antibiotics, decongestants, and phenylephrine, but returned with continued smoking.

Additional evidence of chronic respiratory effects comes from Jamaica, where both heavy marijuana usage and bronchitis are common.[11] However, many Jamaican marijuana users are also heavy tobacco smokers, which clouds the relationship between marijuana and bronchitis. Other studies in Jamaica[12] and Costa Rica[13] found no difference in the incidence of respiratory illness among marijuana smokers and nonsmokers.

A well-controlled study of 74 persons who had smoked marijuana for two to five years found a mild but significant increase in airflow resistance in the large airways, with no effect on conventional pulmonary tests.[14]

Auerbach[15] found evidence of chronic bronchitis among heavy hashish users. Physical examinations revealed abnormal respiratory sounds (rhonchi, wheezes, and rales), though chest X-rays were normal. Lung capacity was 15 to 40 percent below normal, and in 6 of the 20 patients studied, biopsies showed abnormal bronchial tissue resembling that of older heavy tobacco smokers, as well as atypical cells not found in tobacco smokers.

Pulmonary Immune Effects

The effect of marijuana smoke on alveolar macrophages is not clear. In vivo studies using macrophages from rat lungs show a decrease in bactericidal activity,[14-19] but another report[20] shows no significant effect of marijuana smoke (or tobacco smoke) on macrophage activity.

Neoplastic Changes in the Lung

Correlation of marijuana smoking with lung cancer presents difficult methodological problems, because of lung cancer's long latency period, the tendency not to report a history of marijuana use, and the concurrent use of tobacco by many marijuana smokers. Laboratory studies, however, show that elements of marijuana smoke are mutagenic-and, therefore, likely to be carcinogenic.[21-23] In addition, chemical analysis of marijuana smoke reveals many known carcinogens. Delta-9-THC, however, does *not* appear to be mutagenic.[24-25]

Tennant's[26] and Henderson's[10] studies of American service personnel showed numerous cellular abnormalities associated with heavy hashish smoking. These effects were worse among patients who smoked both hashish and tobacco than among those who smoked only tobacco. Thus, the cellular effects of the two substances seem to be additive.

Cardiovascular Effects

Marijuana smoking results in an almost immediate increase in heart rate and blood pressure, which can aggravate existing cardiac insufficiency or hypertension. In healthy young adults, smoking 10 mg of marijuana increases the heart rate by as much as 90 beats per minute; the effect lasts about one hour.[27] This tachycardia seems to result from both parasympathetic and sympathetic stimulation of the cardiac pacemaker.[28–30] However, studies with propranolol have yielded contradictory answers to the question of whether beta-adrenergic stimulation is involved.[28,31–34]

Although cardiac output may increase by as much as 30 percent after smoking marijuana, blood pressure rises only modestly (if at all), indicating decreased peripheral resistance.[35] Large doses of delta-9-THC have resulted in opposite effects, causing a *drop* in systolic and diastolic blood pressure[36] and in heart rate.[37–41] Some degree of tolerance to these hemodynamic effects occurs among chronic users of marijuana. The changes in cardiac function are not permanent; even in long-term users, they can be reversed by cessation of smoking.[38–41]

Coronary Artery Disease

The long-term cardiovascular risks of marijuana are unknown. It is clear, however, that marijuana can aggravate existing heart conditions. It is known to cause changes in the electrocardiogram.[28,42] It increases the work of the heart in ways that are characteristic of stress,[43] and in all probability can trigger arrhythmias or even myocardial infarction in patients suffering from preexisting coronary artery disease. In addition, by dulling the pain of angina, it can cause the patient to delay taking antianginal medications, which can further contribute to cardiac damage.[43] Increased catecholamine levels as a result of marijuana smoking can stimulate myocardial tissue and trigger arrhythmias.[44]

Marijuana also causes postural hypotension, thereby aggravating coronary artery disease or cerebrovascular insufficiency. And marijuana smoke, like tobacco smoke, can cause the formation of carboxyhemoglobin in the bloodstream, thus compromising the blood's oxygen-carrying capacity.[43]

Other Cardiovascular Effects

Chronic administration of large doses of delta-9-THC promotes sodium retention, and leads to increases in body weight and plasma volume.[38-40] The increased plasma volume seems to be caused by the decrease in orthostatic hypertension that occurs with chronic use,[45] but the mechanisms by which delta-9-THC promotes sodium retention are not clear.

Neurologic Effects

The long-term neurologic consequences of marijuana intoxication are unknown. Early studies using pneumoencephalography suggested that long-term marijuana users suffered from cerebral atrophy, but this research suffered from serious methodological and technological limitations and has not been supported by later studies employing better patient selection and computed tomography (CT).[46,47]

One study, in which rhesus monkeys received delta-9-THC over a five-year period, revealed atrophy of the caudate nucleus and frontal portion of the brain, as measured by CT scanning. The authors caution, however, that the implications of these results are uncertain, especially as regards the effects of long-term marijuana use on humans.[48]

Despite anecdotal reports that marijuana induces seizures in patients with preexisting seizure disorders, the bulk of the evidence suggests that this is not the case.[47] In fact, some cannabinoids have been shown to have antiepileptic properties (see Chapter 6).

Reproductive Effects

Male Reproductive System

Marijuana is antiandrogenic, and a number of its constituents, including delta-9-THC, bind to androgen receptors. In addition, marijuana may act on estrogenic receptors.[49] In males, marijuana diminishes testosterone production and inhibits reproductive function.[50] The magnitude and duration of these effects are not well-established. One study of 20 men who used marijuana at least four days a week for six months found lowered testosterone levels.[50] The testosterone levels, though lower than those of controls, were still within normal range in all but two subjects. Levels of follicle-stimulating hormone (FSH) and sperm counts were also lower in marijuana smokers. The results of this study suggested that all these effects were dose dependent.

However, the study did not control for the use of other drugs concurrently with marijuana. Another study involving men in a research ward who smoked government-supplied marijuana found no suppression of plasma testosterone levels.[51] FSH levels and sperm counts were not reported.

Further research has yielded equally inconsistent results. Hembree *et al.* found a decrease in sperm motility, increased numbers of abnormal sperm, and eventually a decline in sperm counts among subjects who received high doses of marijuana for five to six weeks.[52] They concluded, based on this and other evidence, that marijuana interfered with sperm production by acting directly on the seminiferous tubular epithelium, and not by suppressing gonadotropins. A Costa Rican study, by contrast, found no evidence of suppressed testosterone levels among subjects who had regularly smoked marijuana for at least 10 years.[13] Rats exposed to marijuana from a smoke machine for thirty days exhibited lowered sperm counts, but so did rats exposed to smoke that was free of cannabinoids.[53] However, the rats receiving marijuana smoke had an increased number of abnormal sperm forms.

The conclusions that can be drawn from these conflicting studies are at best tentative. Marijuana is antiadrogenic but it is not known whether the effects translate into decreased libido or impaired fertility. Also unknown is the persistence of these effects—whether they resolve spontaneously after discontinuation of marijuana use, and whether tolerance develops with continued use. Although the effects on developing sexual organisms—that is, adolescents—are not known, it is reasonable to assume that they would be more significant, and perhaps long-lasting, than among adults.

Female Reproductive System

Marijuana causes hormonal disruption of the female reproductive cycle. Women who use marijuana four times a week or more have shorter luteal phases, resulting in shorter menstrual cycles. In addition, plasma prolactin levels are elevated and testosterone levels are depressed. Galactorrhea has been reported in as many as 20% of these cases.[54] One study has found impaired fertility among women who use marijuana;[55] however, it suffers from severe methodological flaws and its findings have been challenged.[56] Animal studies, however, show a suppression of ovarian function and interference with gonadotropin and estrogenic activity in females,[57–64] as well as amenorrhea.[65]

Teratogenicity and Effects on Pregnancy

Animal studies—as well as anecdotal evidence—suggests other disturbing effects among chronic users of relatively low doses of marijuana.[66–73] Female monkeys given oral doses of 2.4 mg/kg of delta-9-THC for one to four years showed a subsequent pattern characteristic of high-risk pregnancies, including a higher-than-normal rate of miscarriage and death of offspring in the early postnatal period.[74,75] Fetal anomalies and neonatal deaths are increased by prenatal marijuana use.[81] Moreover, animal studies consistently show that exposure to marijuana during pregnancy causes growth retardation of the fetus. The underlying mechanism seems to include both direct effects on the fetus and suppression of maternal appetite and weight gain.[76,77,78] In addition, marijuana may reduce the fetal blood supply.[82] Also, symptoms consistent with fetal alcohol syndrome have been observed.[79,80] Indeed, fetal alcohol syndrome is five times more likely when the mother is a user of marijuana.[81]

There is some evidence that the use of marijuana close to the delivery date may prolong and complicate labor. Precipitate labor and meconium passage are more frequent in marijuana users than in control groups. However, other studies of women who smoked marijuana but were otherwise enjoyed good health and living conditions showed no significant effects from prenatal marijuana use.[77,78,79,81] It seems reasonable to conclude from these studies that marijuana may exacerbate other risk factors in pregnancy.

THC crosses the placental barrier[77,78,80] and accumulates in mother's milk. Some studies suggest that marijuana use may interfere with lactation and/or diminish the milk supply by inhibiting prolactin secretion.[77,78,80] Rodent studies show significant levels of THC in nursing infants as a result of maternal exposure to THC, and infant monkeys whose mothers are given THC prove to be lethargic and slow to gain weight. One study[73] found a variety of abnormal responses in newborns whose mothers used large amounts of marijuana during pregnancy. These responses included increased startle reflex, tremors, poor self-quieting, and failure to habituate to light. At one month after birth, the visual effects remained in half the infants, and tremors were present in a fourth of them.

Immune Impairment

Animal studies provide evidence that marijuana impairs the immune system.[83] Human studies are more contradictory, but several do demonstrate mild immunologic impairment as a result of marijuana use. The impairment appears to be reversible with cessation of use.[74] In otherwise healthy subjects, this impairment of the immune system is not accompanied by increased susceptibility to infectious disease; a sufficient reservoir of immunity remains to resist infection.[74] However, the impairment may well come into play in patients who are immunocompromised or otherwise at risk of infection. For example, the use of marijuana as an antiemetic for cancer patients is ill-advised in light of the immunosuppressive effects of antineoplastic agents.

In addition, the immunosuppressive effects take on added importance in light of the total picture of marijuana abuse if, for example, marijuana use is part of a pattern of multiple drug use. It would be reasonable to assume that patients who use intravenous drugs along with marijuana might be at increased risk of developing blood-borne infections, including hepatitis. Similarly, the smoking of contaminated marijuana combined with immune system impairment would seem to place users at heightened risk of respiratory infection. Further, long-term immune system impairment is likely to increase the risk of cancer. All of these effects are speculative, but they should be kept in mind by the practitioner who may be seeing chronic marijuana users in clinical practice.

Summary

Marijuana causes a variety of medical problems.
The most pronounced effects are on the respiratory system, and for the most part appear to result from the
direct action of marijuana smoke on lung tissues. These
acute respiratory effects are dose dependent and reversible with cessation of use. In addition, marijuana
smoke is almost certainly carcinogenic, and although the
long-term risk of lung cancer from marijuana smoking
is not established, it is probably similar to the risk from
cigarette smoking. If a patient smokes both cigarettes
and marijuana, we would expect the effects to be additive at least.

Marijuana use—especially chronic use or use by adolescents—also results in systemic effects on the male
and female reproductive system, and in all likelihood
on the immune system as well. It is difficult to estimate
the ultimate course or severity of these systemic effects;
although most seem to resolve spontaneously with cessation of marijuana use, the data are very sparse.

When considered in light of the long-term psychological effects of marijuana use, these medical problems
raise some disturbing issues. Because their signs and
symptoms are subtle and often nonspecific—for in-
stance, the low-normal hormonal levels and marginally
impaired immune responses—they are likely to be overlooked or attributed to other sources. But the clinical
picture of these somatic disturbances may parallel and
reinforce the nonspecific psychological disturbances
that accompany long-term marijuana use. For example,
a patient may present a host of vague complaints—decreased libido, frequent respiratory infections, mild

depression, and sleep disturbances—all of which may be mutually reinforcing and yet difficult to diagnose. In fact, the patient may present an entirely unrelated complaint, without realizing the effect that marijuana use is having on his or her general well-being. In all these cases, a diagnosis of marijuana dependency may easily be overlooked, especially because the clinician has no baseline to compare against the patient's current condition.

For patients presenting with these sorts of nonspecific symptoms, marijuana use should always be considered as an element in the differential diagnosis. Even when other etiologic factors are identified, marijuana use may be a contributing factor. Because the initial symptoms are nonspecific, it may be difficult to show clear improvement resulting from abstention. Even so, abstinence in these cases is more than simply prudent; it is well-justified by the evidence from animal and human studies.

References

1. Anonymous: Effects of marijuana on the respiratory and cardiovascular systems, in Institute of Medicine: *Marijuana and Health*. Washington, DC, National Academy Press, 1982, p.57.
2. Vachon L, FitzGerald MX, Solliday NH, et al: Single-dose effect of marijuana smoke: Bronchial dynamics and respiratory-center sensitivity in normal subjects. *N Engl J Med* 1973;288:985–989.
3. Zwillich CW, Doekel R, Hammill S, Weil JV: The effects of smoked marijuana on metabolism and respiratory control. *Am Rev Respir Dis* 1978;118:885–891.
4. Shapiro BJ, Tashkin DP, Frank IM: Effects of beta-adrenergic blockade and muscarinic stimulation upon cannabis bronchod-

ilation, in Braude MC, Szara S, (eds): *Pharmacology of Marijuana.* New York, Raven, 1976.

5. Tashkin DP, Shapiro BJ, Lee EY, Harper CE: Subacute effects of heavy marijuana smoking pulmonary function in healthy young males. *N Engl J Med* 1976;294:125–129.

6. Hollister LE: Health aspects of cannabis. *Pharmacol Rev* 1986;38(1):11.

7. Kagan SL: Aspergillus: An inhalable contaminant of marijuana. *N Engl J Med* 1981;304:483–484.

8. Schwartz IS: Marijuana and Fungal infection. *Am J Clin Pathol* 1985;84:256.

9. Tennant FS, Preble M, Prendergast TJ, Ventry P: Medical manifestations associated with hashish. *JAMA* 1971;216:1965–1969.

10. Henderson RL, Tennant FS, Guerry R: Respiratory manifestations of hashish smoking. *Arch Otolaryngol* 1972;95:248–251.

11. Hall JAS: *Testimony in marihuana–hashish epidemic hearing of the Committee of the Judiciary U.S. Senate.* Washington, DC, US Government Printing Office, 1975.

12. Rubin V, Comitas L: *Ganja in Jamaica: A medical anthropological study of chronic marijuana use.* The Hague, The Netherlands, Mouton, 1975.

13. Hernandez-Bolanos J, Swenson EW, Coggins WJ: Preservation of pulmonary function in regular, heavy, long-term marijuana smokers. *Am Rev Resp Dis* 1976;113(suppl):100.

14. Tashkin DP, Calvarese BM, Simmons MS, Shapiro BJ: Respiratory status of seventy-four habitual marijuana smokers. *Chest* 1980;78:699–706.

15. Auerbach O, Stout AP, Hammond EC, Garfinkel L: Changes in bronchial epithelium relation to cigarette smoking and in relation to lung cancer. *N Engl J Med* 1961;265:253–267.

16. Huber GL, Simmons GA, McCarthy CR, et al: Depressant effect of marijuana smoke on antibacterial activity of pulmonary alveolar macrophages. *Chest* 1975;68:769–773.

17. Huber GL, Pochay VE, Shea JW, et al: An experimental animal model for quantifying the biologic effects of marijuana on the defense system of the lung, in Nahas GG, Paton WDM, (eds): *Marihuana: Biological Effects. Analysis, Metabolism, Cellular Responses, Reproduction, and Brain.* Oxford, Pergamon, 1979:301–328.

18. Huber GL, Shea JW, Hinds WE, et al: The gas phase of marijuana smoke and intrapulmonary antibacterial defenses. *Bull Eur Physiopath Resp* 1979;15:491–503.
19. Huber GL, Pochay VE, Pereira W, et al: Marijuana, tetrahydrocannabinol, and pulmonary antibacterial defenses. *Chest* 1980;77:403–410.
20. Drath, DB, Shorey JM, Price L, Huber GL: Metabolic and functional characteristics of alveolar macrophages recovered from rats exposed to marijuana smoke. *Infec Immun* 1979;25:268–272.
21. Busch FW, Seid DA, Wei ET: Mutagenic activity of marihuana smoke condensates. *Cancer Letter* 1979;6:319–324.
22. Seid DA, Wei ET: Mutagenic activity of marihuana smoke condensates. *Pharmacologist* 1979;21:204.
23. Wehner FC, Van Rensburg, SJ, Thiel PG: Mutagenicity of marijuana and transkei tobacco smoke condensates in the salmonella/microsome assay. *Mutation Research* 1980;77:135–142.
24. Glatt H, Ohlsson A, Agurell S, Oesch F: Delta-1-tetrahydrocannabinol and 1-alpha, 2-alpha-epoxyhexahydrocannabinol: Mutagenicity investigation in the Ames test. *Mutation Research* 1979;66:329–335.
25. Van Went, GF: Mutagenicity testing of three hallucinogens: LSD, psilocybin and delta-9-THC, using the micronucleus test. *Experientia* 1978;34:324–325.
26. Tennant FS, Guerry RL, Henderson RL: Histopathologic and clinical abnormalities of the respiratory system in chronic hashish smokers. *Substance and Alcohol Misuse* 1980;1:93–100.
27. Anonymous: Effects of marijuana on the respiratory and cardiovascular systems, in Institute of Medicine: *Marijuana and Health*. Washington, DC, National Academy Press, 1982, p. 66.
28. Beaconsfield P, Ginsburg J, Rainsbury R: Marihuana smoking: cardiovascular effects in man and possible mechanisms. *N Engl J Med* 1972;287:209–212.
29. Martz R, Brown DJ, Forney RB, et al: Propranolol antagonism of marihuana-induced tachycardia. *Life Sci* 1972;11:999–1005.
30. Sulkowski A, Vachon L, Rich ES: Propranolol effects on acute marihuana intoxication in man. *Pyschopharmacology* 1977;52:47–53.
31. Bright TP, Kiplinger GF, Brown D, et al: Effects of beta-adrenergic blockade on marijuana-induced tachycardia, in *National*

Academy of Sciences: Report of the 33rd Annual Scientific Meeting of the Committee on Problems of Drug Dependence. Washington, DC, Author, vol. 2, 1971.

32. Perez-Reyes M, Lipton MA, Timmons MC, et al: Pharmacology of orally administered delta-9-tetrahydrocannabinol. *Clin Pharmacol Ther* 1973;14:48–55.

33. Kanakis CJ, Pouget JM, Rosen KM: The effects of delta-9-tetrahydrocannabinol (cannabis) on cardiac performance with and without beta blockage. *Circulation* 1976:53:703–707.

34. Tashkin DP, Soares JR, Hepler RS, Shapiro BJ, Rachelefsky GS: Cannabis 1977. *Ann Intern Med* 1978;89:539–549.

35. Anonymous: Effects of marijuana on the respiratory and cardiovascular systems, in Institute of Medicine: *Marijuana and Health.* Washington, DC, National Academy Press, 1982, p. 67.

36. Kochar MS, Hosko MJ: Electrocardiographic effects of marihuana. *JAMA* 1973;225:25–27.

37. Bernstein JG, Becker D, Babor TF, Mendelson JH: Physiological assessments: cardiopulmonary function, in Mendelson JH, Rossi AM, Meyers RE, (eds): *The Use of Marijuana: A Psychological and Physiological Inquiry.* New York, Plenum Press, 1974.

38. Benowitz NL, Jones RT: Cardiovascular effects of prolonged delta-9-tetrahydrocannabinol ingestion. *Clin Pharmacol Ther* 1975;18:287–297.

39. Benowitz NL, Jones RT: Effects of delta-9-tetrahydrocannabinol on drug distribution and metabolism. *Clin Pharmacol Ther* 1977;22:259–268.

40. Benowitz NL, Jones RT: Prolonged delta-9-tetrahydrocannabinol ingestion: Effects of sympathomimetic amines and autonomic blockades. *Clin Pharmacol Ther* 1977;21:336–342.

41. Nowlan R, Cohen S: Tolerance to marijuana: Heart rate and subjective "high." *Clin Pharmacol Ther* 1977;22:550–556.

42. Johnson S, Domino EF: Some cardiovascular effects of marihuana smoking in normal volunteers. *Clin Pharmacol Ther* 1971;12:762–768.

43. Anonymous: Effects of marijuana on the respiratory and cardiovascular systems, in Institute of Medicine: *Marijuana and Health.* Washington, DC, National Academy Press, 1982, p. 72.

44. Anonymous: Effects of marijuana on the respiratory and car-

diovascular systems, in Institute of Medicine. *Marijuana and Health*. Washington, DC, National Academy Press, 1982, p. 70.

45. Anonymous: Effects of marijuana on the respiratory and cardiovascular systems, in Institute of Medicine: *Marijuana and Health*. Washington, DC, National Academy Press, 1982, p. 69.

46. Campbell, AMG, Evans M, Thomson JLG, Williams MJ: Cerebral atrophy in young cannabis smokers. *Lancet* 1975∞:1219–1225.

47. Anonymous: Effects of marijuana on the brain, in Institute of Medicine: *Marijuana and Health*. Washington, DC, National Academy Press, 1982, p. 87.

48. McGahan J, Dublin A, Sassenrath E. Long-term delta-9-tetrahydrocannabinol treatment. *Am J Dis Child* 1984;138:1109–1112).

49. Purohit V, Ahluwahlia BS, Vigersky RA: Marijuana inhibits dihydrotestosterone binding to the androgen receptor. *Endocrinology* 1980;107:848–850.

50. Kolodny RC, Masters WH, Kolodner RM, Toro G: Depression of plasma testosterone levels after chronic intensive marijuana use. *N Engl J Med* 1974;290:872–874.

51. Mendelson JH, Kuehnle J, Ellingboe J, Babor TF: Plasma testosterone levels before, during, and after chronic marihuana smoking. *N Engl J Med* 1974;291:1051–1055.

52. Hembree WC, Nahas GG, Zeidenberg P, Huang HFS: Changes in human spermatozoa associated with high-dose marihuana smoking, in Nahas GG, Paton WDM, (eds.): *Marihuana: Biological Effects. Analysis, Metabolism, Cellular Responses, Reproduction, and Brain*. Oxford, Pergamon, 1979, pp. 429–439.

53. Huang, HFS, Nahas GG, Hembree WC: Effects of marihuana inhalation on spermatogenesis of the rat, in Nahas GG, Paton WDM, (eds): *Marihuana: Biological Effects. Analysis, Metabolism, Cellular Responses, Reproduction, and Brain*. Oxford, Pergamon, 1979, pp. 419–427.

54. Cohen S: Marijuana and reproductive functions. *Drug Abuse and Alcoholism Newsl* 1985;13:1.

55. Bauman JE, Kolodny RC, Dornbusch RL, Webster SK: Efectos endocrinos del use cronico de la mariguana en mujeres, in *Simposio Internacional Sobre Actualizacion en Mariguana*. Tlalpan, Mexico, July 1979, vol 10, pp. 85–97. [Cited in Institute of Medicine: *Marijuana and Health*. Washington, DC, National Academy Press, 1982, p. 97.

80   Chapter 3

56. Anonymous: Effects of marijuana on the brain, in Institute of Medicine. Marijuana and Health. Washington, DC, National Academy Press, 1982, p. 98.
57. Chakravarty I, Sengupta D, Bhattacharyya, P, Ghosh JJ: Effect of treatment with cannabis extract on the water and glycogen contents of the uterus in normal and estradiol-treated prepubertal rats. Toxicol Appl Pharmacol 1975;34:513–516.
58. Dixit VP, Arya M, Lohiya NK: The effect of chronically administered cannabis extract on the female genital tract of mice and rats. Endokrinologie 1975;66:365–368.
59. Nir I, Ayalon D, Tsafiri A, et al: Suppression of the cyclic surge of luteinizing hormone secretion and of ovulation in the rat by delta-1-tetrhydrocannabinol. Nature 1973;243:470–471.
60. Ayalon D, Nir I, Cordova T, et al: Acute effect of delta-1-tetrahydrocannabinol on the hypothalamo-pituitary-ovarian axis in the rat. Neuroendocrinology 1977;23:31–42.
61. Marks BH: Delta-1-tetrahydrocannabinol and luteinizing hormone secretion. Prog Brain Res 1973;39:331–338.
62. Tyrey L: Delta-9-tetrahydrocannabinol suppression of episodic luteinizing hormone secretion in the ovariectomized rat. Endocrinology 1978;102:1808–1814.
63. Besch NF, Smith CG, Besch PK, Kaufman RH: The effect of marihuana (delta-9-tetrahydrocannabinol) on the secretion of luteinizing hormone in the ovariectomized Rhesus monkey. Am J Obstet Gynecol 1977;128:635–642.
64. Asch RH, Fernandez EO, Smith CG, Pauerstein CJ: Precoital single doses of delta-9-tetrahydrocannabinol block ovulation in the rabbit. Fertil Steril 1979;31:331–334.
65. Asch RH, Smith CG, Siler-Khodr TM, Pauerstein CJ: Effects of delta-9-tetrahydrocannabinol during the follicular phase of the Rhesus monkey (Macaca mulatta). J Clin Endocrin Metab 1981;52:50–55.
66. Braude MC, Ludford JP: Marijuana Effects on the Endocrine and Reproductive Systems. Washington, DC, US Government Printing Office, 1984, pp. 115–123.
67. Anonymous: Effects of marijuana on other biological systems, in Institute of Medicine: Marijuana and Health. Washington, DC, National Academy Press, 1982, p. 99.

68. Gerber WF, Schramm LC: Effect of marihuana extract on fetal hamsters and rabbits. *Toxicol Appl Pharmacol* 1969;14:276–282.
69. Linn S, Schoenbaum SC: The association of marijuana use with outcome of pregnancy. *Am J Public Health* 1983;73:1161.
70. Hingston R, et al: Effects of maternal drinking and marijuana use on fetal growth and development. *Pediatrics* 1982;70:539–546.
71. Abel EL: Prenatal exposure to cannabis: A critical review of effects on growth, development, and behavior. *Behav Neurol Biol* 1980;29:137.
72. Qazi QH, Mariano E, Milman DH, Beller E, Crombleholme W: Abnormalities in offspring associated with prenatal marihuana exposure. *Dev Pharmacol Ther* 1985;8:141–148.
73. Jones KL, Chernoff GF: Effects of chemical and environmental agents, in Creasy RK, Resnik R, (eds): *Maternal Fetal Medicine*. Philadelphia, WB Saunders, 1984.
74. Anonymous: Effects of marijuana on other biological systems, in Institute of Medicine: *Marijuana and Health*. Washington, DC, National Academy Press, 1982, p. 100.
75. Sassenrath EN, Banovitz CA, Chapman LF: Tolerance and reproductive deficit in primates chronically drugged with delta-9-THC. *Pharmacologist* 1979;21:201.
76. Fried PA, Buckingham M, Von Kulmiz P. Marijuana use during pregnancy and prenatal risk factors. *Am J Obstet Gynecol* 1983;146:992–994.
77. Institute of Medicine: *Marijuana and Health*. Washington, DC, National Academy Press, 1982.
78. Pinkert TM (ed): *Current Research on the Consequences of Maternal Drug Abuse*. NIDA Research Monograph 59. Rockville, MD, Department of Health and Human Services, 1985.
79. Braude MC, Ludford JP (eds): *Marijuana Effects on the Endocrine and Reproductive Systems: A RAUS Review Report*. NIDA Research Monograph 44. Rockville, MD, Department of Health and Human Services, 1984.
80. Fehr KO. Kalant H, eds: *Addiction Research Foundation/World Health Organization Meeting on Adverse Health and Behavioral Consequences of Cannabis Use*. Toronto, Addiction Research Foundation, 1983.

81. Marijuana and reproductive functions. *Psych News* 1986 (Sep 19):13.
82. Murthy et al: Long-term effects of marihuana smoke on uterine contractility and tumour development in rats. *West Indian J Med* 1985;34:244.
83. Anonymous: Effects of marijuana on other biological systems, in Institute of Medicine: *Marijuana and Health*. Washington, DC, National Academy Press, 1982, p. 105.

4

Psychiatric Problems Associated with Marijuana Use

A variety of psychiatric reactions are associated with marijuana use. However, a strict cause–effect relationship between marijuana and these reactions does not always exist. Accurate diagnosis and effective treatment must begin with an understanding of the relationship between symptoms and marijuana use.

Predisposing Factors

A number of factors may predispose an individual to psychiatric problems as a result of marijuana use. Two of the most critical are preexisting psychiatric symptoms and the age of insult.[1-3] The younger the age that a person uses marijuana, the greater the likelihood of psychiatric reactions—an alarming fact in light of evidence that marijuana use is being seen in younger and younger populations.[2]

Types of Reactions

Psychiatric symptoms associated with marijuana use fall into the following broad categories: causative, exacerbating, self-medicating, acute, delayed onset, and withdrawal.[4]

Causative

These are symptoms that are caused entirely by cannabis compounds, and that occur even in normal individuals if a high enough dose is taken. They have a rapid onset and are limited in duration. The precise symptoms depend upon the patient and the dose, but typical symptoms were described as early as 1845[1]: euphoria, dissociation of ideas, distortion of time and space; enhancement of hearing; fixed ideas and delusions; damage to the emotions; irresistible impulses; and illusions and hallucinations. Though some of this terminology is rather antiquated, it offers a fair description of symptoms seen today.

Exacerbating

Marijuana use may exacerbate preexisting psychiatric symptoms or may interact with an individual's underlying predisposition. As with causative symptoms, onset is temporally related to marijuana use; however, the symptoms persist beyond the time that the drug is cleared from the system.

Self-Medicating

Some patients with underlying psychiatric disorders may use marijuana because of its perceived antianxiety and antidepressive properties. In reality, however, these effects have not been established—and, indeed, long-term use may actually *worsen* these problems, setting up a cycle that can quickly lead to addiction. For example, individuals may use marijuana in the mistaken belief that it will help them sleep or that it will relieve their depression, but in reality marijuana has been shown to cause insomnia and depression. As symptoms worsen, the individual uses larger and larger doses to try to relieve them, and so on until a compulsive, addictive-use pattern is established.

Acute Reactions

The most frequent adverse reactions to marijuana include severe panic attacks and reactions, and extreme anxiety, usually lasting less than 24 hours.[5-7] Other acute reactions include depression—which may be severe enough to require hospitalization—and acute toxic psychoses, sometimes accompanied by clouding of consciousness.[5,8,9] Toxic psychoses usually have manic or schizoaffective properties, and usually resolve within a few weeks.[5,8] They may, however, be more persistent, and as they become chronic they resemble typical schizophrenia.[5,9] Patients with a history of schizophrenic or manic episodes are at high risk of having active psychosis triggered by the use of cannabis.[1,4] Marijuana has been shown to exacerbate preexisting schizophrenia.[10]

Delayed-Onset Reactions

Lowered testosterone levels from chronic use of marijuana may lead to decreased sex drive, as well as such physical anomalies as decreased sperm counts and motility, and in some cases gynecomastia.[4]

Withdrawal Reactions

Animal and human studies show mild tolerance effects as well as an abstinence syndrome following cessation of marijuana use,[11,12] with symptoms lasting about eight days.

Psychological Problems Associated with Marijuana

Amotivational Syndrome

Controversy exists over the issue of whether chronic marijuana use causes an "amotivational syndrome." Some investigators have identified or postulated such a syndrome, with symptoms including lethargy, diminished scholastic and/or job performance, and introversion. Some, in contrast, have noted symptoms that appear to be contradictory to this clinical picture, with elements of aimless violence and aggression. The common thread in these descriptions seems to be a generalized dysfunction of cognitive, social, and interpersonal skills to a greater or lesser degree.

From a strict scientific viewpoint, the existence or nonexistence of such a syndrome is difficult to establish. Much of the evidence is anecdotal, with many obvious confounding factors. Animal studies of aggression yield results that are contradictory and not easily extrapolated to human populations (see Chapter 2). In addition, the definition of such a "syndrome" is conceptually imprecise.

Though anecdotal, the evidence is strong that many people—especially young people—with drug problems tend to suffer from the sorts of personality dysfunctions that have been included in the term *amotivational syndrome*. Indeed, a new class of psychiatric patient is being identified across the United States—typically young transient males who are prone to depression and anger, who often engage in aggressive, impulsive, and self-destructive acts, and who are uncooperative with treatment.[13] Abuse of drugs, including marijuana, is a virtually universal finding among these patients. However, its precise role in this clinical picture is not at all clear. It may be causative or exacerbating, or it may be a symptom of other underlying causes.

One study shows a relationship between adolescent misbehavior and *subsequent* marijuana use.[14] This study suggests that marijuana use, rather than causing behavioral problems, may be a symptom of an underlying disorder. (See also the discussion on the gateway concept in Chapter 1.) If so, the implication is that certain behavioral problems are indicative of future problems with marijuana. The study used the NIMH Diagnostic Interview Schedule[15] and included factors such as school misbehavior, expulsion, suspension, truancy, fighting in and out of school, running away from home, stealing, lying, vandalism, and juvenile arrests.

Tennant and Groesbeck surveyed 110 heavy cannabis users and found a pattern of apathy and impaired ability to memorize and concentrate—a clinical picture similar to that seen with abuse of tranquilizers.[9] The extent to which these effects can be generalized to a broader "amotivational syndrome" distinct from marijuana's short-term intoxicating effects is unknown.

An Indian study of heavy cannabis users showed no significant differences in IQ scores (as measured by three different tests) between users and nonusers. However, the researchers did find impairment of the ability to perform psychomotor tasks. In addition, standard personality tests demonstrated disabilities in personal, social, and vocational areas, as well as heightened scores on psychoticism and neuroticism scales.[16]

Aggression

Frischknecht reported that cannabis reduces aggressive behavior among normal male laboratory rats.[17] However, he found that among *stressed* animals, marijuana induces aggressive behavior. His study also found that cannabinoids inhibited sexual behavior, an effect that seems to be distinct from its general sedative effects.

Depersonalization

Depersonalization—a subjective feeling of unreality in one's self and/or surroundings—has been reported in conjunction with marijuana use.[18] Because the experience is entirely subjective, it is unmeasureable—

indeed, it is not clear that different patients are describing the same phenomena. Evidence suggests that depersonalization is associated with or may precipitate panic attacks and/or agoraphobia.

References

1. Brill H, Nahas GG: Cannabis intoxication and mental illness, in Nahas GG (ed): *Marijuana in Science and Medicine.* New York, Raven, 1984.
2. MacDonald DI: *Drugs, Drinking, and Adolescents.* Chicago, Yearbook Medical, 1985.
3. MacDonald DI, Newton M: The clinical syndrome of adolescent drug abuse. *Adv Pediatr* 1981;28:1-25.
4. Estroff TW, Gold MS: Psychiatric presentations of marijuana abuse. *Psych Ann* 1986;16:221-224.
5. Knight F. Role of cannabis in psychiatric disturbance. *Ann NY Acad Sci* 1976;282:64-71.
6. Jefferson JW, Marshall JR: *Neuropsychiatric Features of Medical Disorders.* New York, Plenum Press, 1981.
7. Smith DE: Acute and chronic toxicity of marijuana. *J Psychoactive Drugs* 1968;2:37-47.
8. Rottanburg D, Robins AH, Ben-Arie O, et al: Cannabis-associated psychosis with hypomanic features. *Lancet* 1982∞:1364-1366.
9. Tennant FS, Grosebeck CJ: Psychiatric effects of hashish. *Arch Gen Psychiatry* 1972;27:133-136.
10. Negrete JC, Knapp WP, Douglas DE, Smith WB: Cannabis affects the severity of schizophrenic symptoms: Results of a clinical survey. *Psychological Medicine* 1986;16:515-520.
11. Fredericks AB, Benowitz NL: An abstinence syndrome following chronic administration of delta-9-tetrahydrocannabinol in rhesus monkeys. *Psychopharmacology* 1980;71:201-202.
12. Mendelson JH, Mello NK, Lex BW, et al: Marijuana withdrawal syndrome in a woman. *Am J Psychiatry* 1984;141:1289-1290.
13. Schwartz SR, Goldfinger SM: The new chronic patient: Clinical

characteristics of an emerging subgroup. *Hosp Community Psychiatry* 1982;32:470–474.

14. Anthony JC: *Young adult marijuana use in relation to antecedent misbehaviors*. NIDA Research Monograph Series 55. Rockville, MD, 1984:238–244.

15. Robins LN, Helzer JE, Croughan J, Ratcliff K: National Institute of Mental Health Diagnostic Interview Schedule. *Arch Gen Psych* 1981;38:381–389.

16. Varma VK, Malhotra AK, Dang R, Das K, Nehra R: Cannabis and cognitive functions: A prospective study. *Drug Alcohol Depend.* 1988;21:147–152.

17. Frischknecht HR: Effects of cannabis drugs on social behaviour of laboratory rodents. *Progress in Neurobiology* 1984;22:39–58.

18. Moran C: Depersonalization and agoraphobia associated with marijuana use. *Br J Psych* 1985;146:262–267.

5

Diagnosis of Marijuana Dependency

There is a great deal of controversy over the diagnosis of marijuana dependence. Disagreement about how it is diagnosed and treated is widespread. Indeed, many argue against the definition of marijuana dependence *per se* as a primary disease that requires medical intervention.

Despite the vigor with which these questions are debated, they are essentially academic. Marijuana is used by more people today than ever before. Its use has adverse medical and psychosocial consequences. If left untreated, these consequences can and often do progress to more severe conditions. And yet experience has shown that these problems can be prevented, treated, or mitigated—and that the sooner treatment begins, the greater the likelihood of ultimate success. These facts alone offer ample justification for medical intervention.

Marijuana Use and Marijuana Dependence

Not all marijuana use results in dependence; however, medical and psychological problems resulting from marijuana use may develop even if the diagnostic criteria for dependence are not met. Even chronic users may eventually stop using the drug on their own; indeed, recent evidence from Fair Oaks Hospital suggests that some cases of marijuana abuse are age-related and can resolve spontaneously after adolescence. Nevertheless, the short-term use of marijuana can still cause irreversible social, psychiatric, and medical consequences, such as poor academic performance, trauma related to automobile accidents or other types of accidents, and/or criminal charges. It is impossible to predict whether a given case will progress or resolve on its own. For that reason, it is important to treat *all* cases of marijuana use as potentially addictive.

Identifying Marijuana Use

In clinical practice, laboratory tests are normally used to *confirm* a diagnosis of marijuana dependency, but they do little to help the physician arrive at the diagnosis. Under ordinary circumstances, they would not be ordered unless the practitioner first has some index of suspicion that the patient is using marijuana.

Unfortunately, marijuana dependency may masquerade as a wide variety of complaints. Most of them are nonspecific—sleeplessness, depression that may range from mild to severe, difficulties in school or at work, impaired social functioning, and so on. Often the patient will not volunteer that he or she uses marijuana. Indeed, it may even be denied. In the absence of a reported history of marijuana use and specific symptoms, marijuana dependency may be easily overlooked.

Adding to the difficulty of diagnosis is the fact that the DSM-III-R (*Diagnostic and Statistical Manual of Disorders*, Third edition, revised) criteria for diagnosis of substance abuse are largely irrelevant for diagnosing marijuana dependency. DSM-III-R establishes three requirements for a diagnosis of substance abuse:

- A pattern of pathological use
- Impairment in social or occupational functioning due to substance abuse
- A duration of at least one month

These rigid criteria do not adequately reflect the realities of marijuana dependence, which often has an insidious onset. If one waits for a patient—especially an adolescent patient—to fulfill the DSM-III-R criteria before making a diagnosis, one may be risking the patient's normal development, or even his or her life. Marijuana dependency is extremely difficult to treat successfully, and treatment must begin as early as possible.

Further, the DSM-III-R criteria are controversial because of their subjectivity. Various practitioners interpret them far differently; to one, a minor drop in grades and arguments with friends and family may constitute impairment in social and occupational functioning, whereas to another they may simply be manifestations of the stresses of adolescence.

Schwartz and Hawks have proposed, in lieu of rigid

TABLE 5. Signs and Symptoms Suggestive of
Marijuana Use[a]

Behavioral signs
— Memory problems
    Chronic lying about whereabouts
    Sudden disappearance of money or valuables from the home
    Suspicious robbery or breaking and entering while family is away
— Rapid mood changes
— Abusive behavior toward self or others
—Panic attacks
— Frequent outbursts
— Hostility with lack of insight or remorse
— Increasing secretiveness

Social signs
    Loss of driver's license
    Driving while impaired
    Auto accidents
    Frequent truancy
    Loss of part-time job or problems on the job
    Underachievement over the past 6–12 months
— Definite deterioration of academic or job-related performance
— Dropping out from rigorous sport or other activities
— Legal problems, especially when they involve loss of control—
    e.g., assaults, thefts, disorderly conduct

Circumstantial evidence
    Smell of marijuana on clothes
    Use of drug jargon
    Drug or drug paraphernalia found in room, clothes, or automobile
    Whereabouts unknown for more than 36 hours
    Drug terminology in school notebooks or in yearbook inscriptions
    Change in friends
— Definitive change in peer group preference to peers who are un-
    motivated or who are known users of marijuana
— Change in hygiene or attire

TABLE 5. (cont.)

Medical symptoms
— Chronic fatigue and lethargy
 Chronic nausea or vomiting
 Chronic dry irritating cough
 Chronic sore throat
 Chronic unexplained conjunctivitis
 Chronic bronchitis
 Headaches
— Impaired motor skill coordination
 Trauma—especially repeated trauma

[a] Adapted from Gold MS, Washton AM, Dackis CA, Chatlos JC. New treatments for opiate and cocaine users: But what about marijuana? *Psych Ann* 1986; 16(4):206–212.

diagnostic criteria, the use of descriptive features to identify patients who should undergo urine testing.[1] Similarly, the Fair Oaks Hospital Drug and Rehabilitation Program has developed a series of behavioral, social, and medical cues to alert the physician to ask more questions and order laboratory tests (Table 5).

Some would object that these signs and symptoms could be the result of many factors other than marijuana dependency. We agree; they are simply warning signs that should alert the physician to probe more deeply, and should be seen as suggestive rather than conclusive.

Nonetheless, in light of the ultimate consequences of marijuana dependency—and especially its potential, if ignored, to progress to more serious forms of substance abuse—it is better to err on the side of caution when making a diagnosis. A relatively low "diagnostic

threshold"—with subsequent laboratory confirmation—allows early identification of problems such as
diminished school performance, memory or concentration impairment, loss of motivation, and disruption of
family dynamics. With early intervention, these problems can be addressed before they result in lifelong
consequences.

Distinguishing Cause and Effect

The most important element in diagnosing marijuana addiction is an impairment of the patient's ability
to function, either psychologically or physiologically.[2,3]
However, it is sometimes difficult to establish this
link, because the patient often believes marijuana use
to be a *consequence* of the problem rather than the *cause*
of it.[2,4–6] For example, the patient may suffer from insomnia and believes that he or she uses marijuana to assist
in falling asleep. However, THC suppresses REM sleep,
so it is likely that the patient's sleep disturbances are
themselves caused by the marijuana use.[2,7] Similarly,
patients often cite depression as a reason for their marijuana use, without realizing that depression is a common *consequence* of marijuana use.[7,8]

Interestingly, studies reveal that individuals who
are depressed *initially* do not necessarily use more marijuana as a result.[2] In fact, they may actually use less.
Marijuana addicts, by contrast, appear to use the drug
in spite of worsening depression, even though they
often report a dysphoric response to marijuana inhalation or ingestion.[2,5,9,11]

Confirming the Diagnosis

Laboratory tests can confirm recent marijuana use, and the foregoing factors may be strongly suggestive of addiction, but the diagnosis must be confirmed by identifying the essential features of addiction. It is important, but difficult, to distinguish between *incidental* and *addictive* marijuana use. Not all marijuana use is addictive. For example, there is evidence to suggest that some people may be motivated to use marijuana in response to stress and related problems. But marijuana use in this setting cannot be considered addictive unless it is marked by the behaviors of addiction as described below. Those suffering from marijuana addiction may begin using marijuana in response to stress, but the pattern of use quickly becomes compulsive. In short, addicts are abnormally susceptible to the drug's reinforcing effects—a predisposition that may be inherited.[11–13]

This distinction between incidental and addictive use is difficult to draw conceptually, but is fairly obvious in clinical practice. It is essentially the same distinction as is seen between occasional tranquilizer use and addiction or between alcohol use and alcoholism. Even though the alcoholic may, in the short term, be able to compensate for his or her alcohol use, a careful history will usually reveal compulsive alcohol-related behavior that is absent with the incidental user. Similarly, these *behaviors of addiction* are a reliable and consistent means of diagnosing marijuana addiction. A preoccupation with acquisition, compulsive use, and relapse are the most sensitive indicators that marijuana is a consistent problem of central importance.[2,10,14] Once a personal or social impairment is determined in the setting of active marijuana use, the diagnosis of addictive use can be made.[4,14,15] Preoccupation with marijuana may be manifest in any number of ways, but a common element is the persistent presence of marijuana in the patient's pattern of living and repertoire of choices. Despite problems caused by its use, marijuana will occupy a high priority in the individual's life.[16] Compulsivity is manifest by continued use despite marijuana-related adverse consequences. Regular or repetitive use is a frequent but not essential finding. The key feature is the continued use of marijuana when common sense or logic would dictate moderation or abstinence—for example, continued smoking despite a respiratory infection, or use of marijuana in spite of the danger of legal consequences or loss of one's job.

Additional Considerations

Other Drug Dependencies

An additional signal is a history of other addictive behaviors—especially other drug dependencies. Concurrent drug or alcohol problems are common among patients suffering from marijuana dependency. Frequently a daily marijuana habit is combined with daily or intermittent addictive use of cocaine or alcohol. In fact, multiple addiction is more common than isolated addictions, especially among younger addicts.[4,17] Unfortunately, the patient has the same motivations of denial and deception wherein these drugs are concerned, so the physician must probe carefully and thoroughly during the history.

Tolerance and Physical Dependence

Unlike some other addictions, tolerance and physical dependence are not essential features of the diagnosis. These adaptive mechanisms probably occur in most chronic users whether they are addicted or not, and they vary according to individual factors.[9,16,18] *Tolerance* is often subtle, and may be manifest as mood changes, tachycardia, orthostatic hypotension, skin and body temperature changes, a decrease in intraocular pressure, and slowing of electroencephalograph (EEG) waves and psychomotor task performance.[16] *Dependence* may result in a number of withdrawal symptoms after cessation of marijuana use, including anxiety, depression, sleep and appetite disturbances, irritability, tremors, diaphoresis, nausea, muscle convulsions, and restlessness.[16]

The signs and symptoms of tolerance and dependence may persist for months, because THC is taken up and stored in fat tissues and released slowly into the bloodstream over a long period of time. In addition, the subtlety of these signs and symptoms make them easy to overlook or attribute to other causes. Thus, their use in diagnosis is questionable at best.[16]

Denial

As with all addictions, denial is a common and essential feature of marijuana addiction. Often it is not limited to the patient, but is also found among family members, friends, and co-workers. This denial complicates both diagnosis and treatment, and it requires a departure from the traditional one-to-one patient–physician assessment. Obviously the history-taking should involve the patient's family and others, but the physician must be prepared for denial, noncooperation, or even outright hostility on their part.

Case Reports: The Diagnosis of Marijuana Abuse

Case 1: K.

This was an emergency, voluntary admission for this 16-year-old white, single male. This is K.'s second psychiatric hospitalization and first Fair Oaks admission. K. lives with his family of origin, which includes his mother, age 46, a homemaker who completed 2 years of college; his father, age 49, an investment banker; and brother, age 11, who is in the sixth grade. There are three brothers living outside the family home: One is a computer analyst living in Paris; another, age 24, is an investment banker, and the other, age 23, is also an investment banker. K. is currently in the tenth grade in public school, classified perceptually impaired and attending a supplemental class. He is unemployed.

Chief Complaint

"Fighting with my parents constantly about their rules."

History of the Present Illness

K. reported going home for one day in order to celebrate his birthday after discharge from another hospital. He was admitted there in January after an altercation with his father in which he threatened to stab him. K. stated for the past 4½ years he has become increasingly oppositional, refusing to obey parents' rules. His identified negative behavior coincides with his use of marijuana that he abruptly stopped December 30, 1985, because he became aware that his memory had deteriorated. He stated that he attended Narcotics Anonymous meetings for support and received additional support from his friends and girlfriend who have continued their marijuana use. K. thought his bad attitude would dissipate when he stopped marijuana; however, this did not occur. He reported 1 month prior to admission that his father smacked him "on reflex" when K. called his mother a bad name. Ever since that episode, K. had been trying to provoke father with plans to hit his father back if his father were to initiate physical contact.

K. reported that before marijuana use he had temper tantrums consisting of crying, throwing things, and punching walls. While at another hospital, K. went into the quiet room and punched walls for half an hour after breaking up with his girlfriend.

K. stated his mood varies. When he is upset, he finds it hard to eat. Sleep, energy, and concentration problems were denied.

K. reported awareness of learning problems since the fourth grade when the family moved from Virginia to New Jersey. He stated he went from a high reading group to the lowest reading group and had difficulty understanding mathematical concepts. He was classified perceptually impaired by the child study team in 1985.

Records from St. Clare's Hospital indicate K. became easily angered, frustrated, and was generally oppositional. While on a pass, K. and his parents engaged in a verbal power struggle about K.'s haircut, to the point that they could not spend time together.

Parents provided more information, stating that 1½ years ago they noticed K. began rebelling against rules. At that time, he would create "scenes" with scheming, throwing things, and pushing his father. He had changed his group of

friends to drug-using peers, and his parents found para-
phernalia, including a water pipe, in his possession. Two
days prior to the first admission, his parents reported K.
threatened to kill his father, told his brother that he would
beat him up if he had him alone, and threatened to kill his
mother. His parents called the police who spoke to K. As his
behavior continued to escalate, the following night police at
his parent's request brought K. to a psychiatric hospital. K.
was treated briefly with nortriptyline 10 mg that was discontinued as K. felt giddy.

His parents reported K. began seeing a psychologist for
six sessions in the summer of 1984. Contact was initiated as
K. was saying to his parents, "I want to die." He later told
his parents that he said this because he was angry. For the
past 4 to 5 months, K. had been seen by a psychologist. His
family was seen once a week, and K. was seen individually
once a week.

Past Psychiatric History

Included in history of the present illness.

Medical History

K. reported having chickenpox without sequelae. He had
pneumonia at age 11. High prolonged fevers, headaches, and
seizures were denied. K. stated he has had minor sports injuries without requiring medical treatment. His mother reported that K. was accident-prone as a young child and had
many injuries requiring sutures. He fractured his right wrist
twice. At age 10, he fell while ice skating, lost consciousness
briefly, and had concussive symptoms without sequelae. Surgery was denied. There is a hearing loss in the left ear from
repeated ear infections. K. reported being farsighted and
stated he was supposed to wear glasses for reading. His

weight has been maintained at a 144 lb at 5'11" tall. K. reported beginning smoking cigarettes at age 13 and currently smokes one pack per day. He drinks one beer every 4 months.

His mother reported K. had severe milk allergies as an infant, resulting in rash and milk intolerance. In addition, he is allergic to mold, dust, and pollen and received desensitization seasonally.

Family Medical and Psychiatric History

One brother had Osgood Schlatter's disease. Another has hypertension. A maternal aunt had died at age 33 from colon cancer. His maternal grandmother died at age 56 from atherosclerosis in 1984. His maternal grandfather died during surgery for ligation of veins. His father has a history of hypertension and Osgood Schlatter's disease. His paternal uncle died from a heart attack at age 45. His paternal grandfather died from leukemia at age 73. A maternal relative had a history of goiter. One brother has had reading difficulties.

Psychosocial and Developmental History

K. is the next to youngest brother born to a middle-class family of Irish and English descent. His father was in the Navy until he retired and pursued his present occupation. While in the Navy, he was intermittently absent due to assignments at sea. K. stated he was closest to his oldest brother. He stated both brothers remained in college for more than 4 years, and his parents seemed supportive of this. His parents view K. as competitive with his older brothers. K. has lived at home with the exception of 1 summer when he worked as kitchen help at a camp.

A significant loss is his brother's moving to Paris. K. stated he and his brother were similar in that they did not get along with their parents. His parents also felt that significant losses included his maternal grandparent's death, paternal grandfather's death, and the death of the pastor of their church in 1980.

K. stated he was raised in the Catholic religion and, at this point, would like to attend church. K. stated in the past he rejected religion.

His mother reported bleeding in the first trimester of pregnancy with K. His birth weight was 8 lb, 10 oz. Labor and delivery were essentially within normal limits. The milk allergy was described previously. The neonatal period was characterized by vomiting, colic, and sleep disturbance. Early childhood behaviors were characterized by overactivity, inability to sit still, being fidgety, inability to tolerate delay, impulsivity, difficulty accepting correction, temper tantrums, unresponsive to discipline, failure to complete projects, feeling left out, withdrawing, accident prone, demanding attention and affection, not working up to ability, and being easily frustrated. His mother reported developmental milestones were achieved within normal limits with walking occurring at age 15½ months. K. was toilet trained at 2½ years. His mother cannot recall when language skills were acquired. K. described being successful in sports, particularly lacrosse and soccer. He was able to ride a two-wheeler bicycle at 5. Letter reversal was denied.

His mother reported K. had trouble learning colors and was older than the other children when he finally mastered this skill. He attended public school for kindergarten and first grade. Toward the end of the first grade, K. began having difficulty with mathematics. His parents moved him to a private Catholic school for 1 year, and K.'s grades improved. The family moved to New Jersey when his father retired from the Navy, and K. attended public schools from fourth grade on. He received C's and D's, and teachers always felt he would do better if he worked harder. K. reported to his parents that he had given up trying in the sixth grade. K. was first worked up by the child-study team in the eighth grade, and he was placed in supplemental training.

K. reported in the sixth and seventh grades that he was suspended, once for fighting and once for writing a word in a friend's yearbook. In the eighth grade, he was suspended for smoking on school premises. Bizarre, habitual behaviors, head banging and rocking, fire setting, enuresis, cruelty to animals, and school truancy were denied. K. also denied vandalism. He stated he has taken money from his mother's purse but denied other stealing behavior. He ran away twice, sleeping over at friends' homes because of fighting with his parents. He had gotten into a fight with another boy over his girlfriend. He stated he was hit, and he fought back. Legal difficulties were denied.

K. expressed interest in carpentry and hoped to pursue this as a career. Military history was denied.

Description of Current Family Issues/Dynamics

Mr. and Mrs. L. describe a stable cohesive family with predominantly positive relationships among members. Except for K.'s current difficulties, problematic issues in the family are denied. However, his parents relate that K. has always compared himself unfavorably with the three older brothers. They are reportedly close to each other and are seen as doing well in their careers at this time. His parents describe attempting to reassure K. that he did not have to compare himself to the older brothers but see this as unsuccessful.

His younger brother B. is reported to have a learning disability. Behavior problems have been minimal in this child, according to parents.

K. and the father are described as having a history of closeness. However, K. seemed to his parents to have felt rejected by curtailing of their outings together due to his parents' feeling the need to cut back financially. Since November

1985, according to his parents, when his father uncharacter-istically hit him, K. has been perceived to be angry at him. He seems to parents to attempt to goad the father into hitting him again so he can strike back. Mr. L. has felt in good control and has not been provoked at this point. He describes K. as close to his mother and as confiding in her. Mr. and Mrs. L. see K.'s drug problem as a symptom of an underlying prob-lem focusing here as his perceived low self-esteem and learn-ing disability. They much question the need for continued inpatient hospitalization. They express much concern that the deprivations they perceive K. to experience on the unit will undermine what they see as his current motivation to stop drug use.

His parents are remaining in close contact with K. during the hospitalization. They relate that, although the brothers have been angry with him for upsetting the family, they are working this through and offering K. support.

His parents have agreed to K.'s staying in the hospital long enough to complete the evaluation and state they will then consider if he should stay for treatment.

Mental Status Examination

K. presented as a neatly groomed male appearing his stated age of 16. He assumed a seated position, and eye con-tact was established and maintained. Facial expression was mobile and congruent with his dysphoric mood. Affect was appropriate to thought content and demonstrated full range. Speech was of normal tone and somewhat underproductive. No speech impediments were apparent. Thoughts were log-ical, abstract, and coherent. At the time of interview, hallu-cinations, delusions, déjà vu, phobias, compulsions, deper-sonalization, derealization, and suicidal homicidal ideation were denied. K. reported previously feeling that he wanted to physically attack his father and had made attempts to pro-voke his father to hit him first.

On formal testing, K. was oriented in three spheres. The fund of knowledge was good. Remote and recent memory appeared unimpaired. Serial 7s were performed with one error as were serial 3s. Digit span was 6 forward and 4 in reverse. Similarities and proverbs were abstracted adequately. Judgment was impaired and demonstrated lack of social responsibility as K. would do "nothing" if he lost a book belonging to the library, and, if he saw a letter on the street, he would "leave it there." K.'s three wishes were that "my parents and I never fight again, that I could be rich, and I would always be happy." He would like to be a "squirrel as they lead a simple life." He wishes to "change my temper." In 5 years he saw himself in college.

Admitting Diagnosis

- Axis I   Cannabis abuse
              Conduct disorder
- Axis II   Deferred
- Axis III   None

Physical and Neurological Examination

Physical examination revealed a height of 5'11", weight 144 lb, blood pressure 128/86, temperature 98.7, pulse 130, and respiration 20. The remainder of the physical examination was unremarkable, including a normal HEENT examination, nonpalpable thyroid, normal cardiovascular, and pulmonary exam, and a normal abdominal examination. Impression was of a normal physical examination. The neurological examination revealed intact cranial nerves, no focal neurological signs, normal sensory and motor function, reflexes were symmetrical and hyperactive, and there were no signs of abnormal gait or coordination. The impression was that of a normal neurological examination.

Laboratory Findings

On admission, patient had a normal CBC with differential, RPR, ESR, urinalysis, chest X-ray, and EKG with a rate of 97 beats per minute. A SMA 22 was normal, except for elevated triglycerides of 252, and an elevated glucose of 122, with a subsequent fasting glucose of 102. The comprehensive drug evaluation on admission was negative for all drugs, including cannabinoids. Neuroendocrine testing revealed a normal pattern of diurnal cortisol testing, and a DST of 7 points revealed no evidence of nonsuppression or depression. A sleep-deprived EEG with NP leads was negative, and an echocardiogram evaluation was WNL without evidence of mitral valve prolapse or other valve dysfunction. An X-ray of both hands revealed no abnormalities and was ordered after the patient hit the wall and had swollen his hand. On the treatment unit, several adolescent drug screens of urine were negative for all drugs tested.

Psychological Testing

The WAIS-R showed a Verbal IQ of 100, Performance IQ of 102, and a Full Scale IQ of 102. The WRAT scores revealed a reading level in the 70th percentile, spelling 47th percentile, and arithmetic at 58th percentile. There was mild difficulty with visual motor integration, and some soft neurological signs. He was unable to depict three-dimensional figures, and his performance on the Benton Test was mildly impaired because of difficulty reproducing some of the more complex drawings. Nonverbal short-term memory was WNL. There was some evidence of mild concentration difficulties. Tests findings are consistent with probably mild long-standing developmental dysfunction such as attention deficit disorder. His current achievement testing results suggested he has acquired basic academic skills. The aforementioned areas of impairment or weakness may continue to impede his performance in school, and continued supplemental academic help in school as well as psychological intervention is recommended. On personality testing, there was some evidence of mild organicity on the Bender Gestalt, as well as evidence of an adjustment disorder with depressed mood. There was no evidence of structural disorganization and no evidence of schizophrenia, psychosis, or borderline pathology. K.'s temper outbursts seemed to have been the result of buildup of stress that severely altered his ability to maintain adequate control. K. has a low self-image, feels isolated and frightened of the future.

Consultations

None.

Interim Diagnosis

- Axis I   Cannabis abuse, continuous oppositional disorder, attention deficit disorder, residual type
- Axis II   Deferred
- Axis III   Hearing loss left ear

Initial Formulation

K. presents with an 18-month history of marijuana abuse and oppositional behavior. This behavior is superimposed on a longer standing problem with attention, concentration, and frustration tolerance. His history indicates an attention deficit disorder with residual hyperactivity characterized by early sleep difficulties, feeding difficulties, hyperactivity, poor attention, impulsivity, and not being responsive to discipline. Substance abuse and acting out seem concurrent with K.'s classification of perceptual impairment and the introduction of remediation through a supplemental room in school. It is unclear how this process was interpreted by K.; however, in this achievement-oriented family, K. may have experienced significant decrease in self-esteem. In an attempt to gain control, his parents tend to overreact and argue with K. about many details. There is a long-standing hearing deficit in the left ear secondary to chronic ear infections as a young child.

Counselor's Course in Treatment

Upon admission to ACCEPT Unit, patient was hostile and resistant to treatment. The patient initially signed a 72-hour notice and threatened to leave treatment. The patient had to be seen with his family to resolve conflict of his wanting to leave treatment. After discussion with his parents, the patient decided to withdraw the 72-hour notice and commit himself to completing inpatient treatment. Although the patient withdrew the 72-hour notice, he continued to show and verbalize resistance to treatment and being involved in interacting with peers and staff. Patient also exhibited an anxiety in dealing with any of his own issues and feelings and verbalizing issues around conflicts with him and his parents.

The patient frequently had conflicts with other peers and at times would be sadistic and verbally abusive to peers and staff. Patient admitted to feelings of fear and rejection or being close with other peers and verbalized that he had always been a loner and always felt rejected by others. Patient was able to work through this conflict and improved his interactions with peers and staff.

On March 20, 1986, patient was able to achieve Status I and verbalized admittance of his powerlessness over his chemical dependency and the need to work on his recovery from his chemical dependency. The patient exhibited defensiveness of anger and fear of taking Step I. On April 12, 1986, patient achieved Status II after being able to verbalize desire to be restored to sanity by a power greater than himself. The patient showed extreme difficulty in taking the step in acknowledging the need for him to become aware of his negative behavior toward others. He got in touch with feelings of hate and self-worthlessness. Patient was able to achieve Status III on May 10, 1986, after being able to verbalize a desire to work Step III and to turn his life over to a power greater than himself. Patient completed his Step IV on June 2, 1986, and presented his Step IV to Joel Warner, a clergyperson, on June 6, 1986. Patient participated in family intervention on March 13, 1986, and dealt with parents' feelings of anger and hurt over patient's behavior while he was using drugs and alcohol. Patient exhibited feelings of anger and distance toward his parents and younger brother who attended intervention. Patient attended family week from April 14 to April 18, 1986. Patient was able to deal with conflict toward himself and his mother and father and feelings of rejection by his older brothers. A series of family sessions were held after family week in order that the patient and father could deal with their conflicts. Patient was able to acknowledge feelings of hatred, and his father was able to acknowledge feelings of hurt and betrayal by the patient; as a result, patient and father were able to work out severe conflicts in their relationship by the end of treatment. Patient's mother was able to work on detaching herself from her son's behavior and gain awareness of her own codependency over her son.

Treatment Plans and Goals

1. For patient to gain awareness of his chemical dependency and verbalize commitment to a drug-free lifestyle.
2. For patient to gain awareness of his oppositional behavior on the unit and to participate in all activities as a result of his awareness.

3. For patient to become aware of his family dysfunction and demonstrate appropriate behavior and verbalize feelings with family members.

Course in Hospital

Medical. During the evaluation period, K. developed tonsillitis and was treated with Penicillin VK 250 mg QID for 10 days. During the treatment portion, patient hit his hand against the wall, had some swelling, but an X ray revealed no evidence of bony abnormality. During the hospitalization, patient was treated with Retin A for a mild case of acne with good resolution during treatment. He participated well in the exercise program and improved his overall fitness during hospitalization.

Psychiatric. During the evaluation period, patient was resistant to treatment, often remaining superficial and projecting anger toward the staff. Parents would promise gifts and trips if he remained in the hospital. On transfer to the treatment unit, patient clearly stated that he did not want to be in the program. Following a period of superficiality, there was further joining with the group with expressions of homesickness and sadness that were verbalized as his behavior was compliant. There was development of an ambivalent attitude and irritability with an attitude of arrogance as patient did not feel that he fit in with his peers. The irritability persisted as the focus more clearly became on family issues. There was a development of opposition to authority that continued as a major focus throughout his treatment. Family week assisted in engaging the family much more directly in the treatment and assistance in K.'s progress. The oppositional aspects of his personality problems persisted throughout treatment but were addressed repeatedly. There was significant fear of physical damage related to fighting in the family. There was anger mobilized as the patient was interrupted or "cut off" during therapy sessions. When this was confronted, issues of trust, loneliness, and rejection became clear. There were sadistic expressions of anger toward peers, staff, and parents that were focused on with some resolution. By the end of treatment, patient became a role model in the community, was able to focus on and express intense affects with full control. During termination, patient could express sadness and focus on feelings of missing peers as well as fears of approaching discharge. During the hospitalization, there was no evidence of psychosis or major depression, and patient was not treated with any psychotropic medications.

Condition upon Discharge

Medical. Patient was discharged with no medical problems, with resolution of acne, and was on no medications.

Psychiatric. Upon discharge, patient was not depressed, suicidal, or homicidal. Many aspects of his oppositional disorder were resolved during treatment though minor aspects remained to be focused on in aftercare. There was no evidence of depression upon discharge, and there was much better adjustment to changing conditions in the new situation. Patient was discharged on no medications.

Recommendations and Disposition

1. Patient attend day treatment for 2 weeks upon completion from inpatient treatment.
2. Upon completion of day treatment, patient to be transferred to CLEAN Teens outpatient program at Fair Oaks Hospital.
3. Family members to attend multifamily group in CLEAN Teens Program.

4. Patient attend NA/AA at least five times per week.
5. Family members attend Alanon.

Final Diagnosis

- Axis I   Cannabis abuse, continuous oppositional
              disorder, attention deficit disorder, re-
              sidual parent–child problem, adjust-
              ment disorder with depressed mood
- Axis II   None
- Axis III   Hearing loss left ear, tonsillitis

Case 2: J.

This was an emergency voluntary admission for this 16-year-old, white, single male. This is J.'s first Fair Oaks hospitalization and first psychiatric hospitalization. J. is currently living with his mother, age 47, who is a secretary, and his father, age 51, who is an electrician. J.'s sister, age 26, is an occupational therapist living in Connecticut, and his brother, age 22, owns his own towing business. J. is currently in a work–study program in the eleventh grade. He is currently working at a gas station as a gas station attendant. There is no history of a child study team evaluation having been done.

Chief Complaint

"I'm here for drugs."

History of the Present Illness

J. reports the onset of his current symptoms as March 1986 when he was thrown out of school "because I cut classes all the time." He described that all of his friends cut school, and therefore he just went along with the group. He reported that his drug use began at age 14 when he began using marijuana up to ⅛ ounce per week, and he also began drinking 8 to 10 nips of beer per week every 2 weeks. He also reportedly used mescaline four times in the past year as well as experimenting with cocaine. J. reports that he does not know why he began using drugs and that his friends were using drugs and he felt he wanted to go along with the crowd.

J. also described a current stressor as fighting with his mother. He described that their fighting had increased recently and that this was most problematic for him. He reported that he is closer to his mother than his father, and he supposes that this is why they fight so much. J. also reported that he sold his motorbike and took money out of the bank for drugs. He reported that it was when he sold his motorbike that his parents knew he had a drug problem as his motorbike was his prize possession. He reported that his parents wanted him to come into the hospital as they felt his drug problem was just beginning and could only get worse. He reported that his parents called Fair Oaks, and he was subsequently admitted.

Past Psychiatric History

J. denied past inpatient psychiatric hospitalization as well as outpatient treatment. J. also described the use of psychotropic, antianxiety, or antidepressant medications. Drug use and alcohol use were described in the history of the present illness. There is no further past psychiatric history reported.

Medical History

J. reported that he has had chickenpox; however, he denied having had the measles or the mumps. High prolonged fevers, headaches, head injuries with loss of consciousness, and seizures were denied. J. denied having been in accidents or having any trauma to himself. Medical hospitalization as well as surgical procedures were denied. Venereal disease and thyroid disease as well as hepatitis were denied. Speech and hearing difficulties were denied. J. reportedly wears glasses as he is nearsighted; otherwise he denies any other visual difficulties. J. reported that he has a good appetite and eats three meals a day along with snacking. He reportedly has not gained or lost weight in the recent year. J. reportedly has smoked one half a pack of cigarettes per day for the past 2 years. Allergies to food, medication, or contact were denied. There is no further medical history given by either parents or J.

Family Medical and Psychiatric History

Two maternal uncles have a history of alcohol abuse. J.'s father and brother have a history of alcohol abuse, although the family does not see this as problematic. The paternal grandmother died of a myocardial infarction. There is no further family medical or psychiatric history reported.

Psychosocial and Developmental History

J. is the youngest of three children born to this intact family. J.'s religion is Catholic, and he describes his religion as unimportant to him at this time. J. reported that his ethnicity is Slavic.

Mother reported that her pregnancy history with J. was unremarkable. She reported him to be a good baby to take care of who reached his developmental milestones at age-appropriate times. He reportedly sat without help at 6 months, was toilet trained by 2½ years, and his mother was unable to remember when J. first spoke.

His mother reported that J. was always a shy child; however, that he later had much daredevil behavior. Left to right discrimination was denied, and J. reported that he is right-handed. He reported that he is very good at sports and has had no difficulties with fine or gross motor coordination. There is no history of enuresis, fire setting, or cruelty to animals reported by either J. or his parents. His mother reported that J. has a somewhat short attention span; however, she denied impulsivity or difficulty tolerating delay. His mother described that he is a daydreamer and is involved in lying and stealing. Temper tantrums were denied. Vandalism and truancy were reported by parents. J. also reported truancy and stealing. J. himself reported that he has a somewhat difficult time concentrating; however he is not clear on why this is so.

J. was very vague about his relationship with his parents. He reported having a good relationship with his family and reported them as happy and that they related well with each other. He describes his parents as equal disciplinarians and described getting along well with his sister and brother. J. was unable to give other details concerning his family functioning, although he did report that the fighting with his mother was upsetting to him.

School history was described by J. He reported that he has always had a B/C average and that he did well in science and math. He reported that his grades were better during grammar school than in high school. In high school, he reported repeating the eleventh grade and that he will start the twelfth grade in the fall. He described currently being involved in a work–study school program. There are no further details concerning J.'s school history at this time. Special class placements as well as developmental abilities were denied. J. is currently expelled from school because of truancy.

J. reported that he has been in several incidents of truancy from school as well as stealing and breaking and entry. He reportedly went into his home unbeknown to his parents and took earrings from his mother to buy marijuana. Vandalism was reported by parents, although they did not give details concerning this. Running away, physical fighting, and assault were denied. Legal problems and pending court dates were also denied. There were no detention placements noted.

J. reported that he has always had many friends. He reported that he had a girlfriend as early as age 12 and was sexually active at that time. Homosexual or incestuous relationships were denied. J. described himself as a follower who liked to go along with his peer group.

J. reported many activities, sports, and hobbies that he enjoys. He reported that he enjoys skateboarding, swimming, riding his dirtbike, playing hackeysack, unicycle riding, taking care of his tropical fish, and playing tennis and football. He reported that he would like to race dirtbikes when he gets older or fix boats or work in real estate. He is currently working as a gas station attendant.

Military history was denied.

Legal history was denied.

Description of Current Family Issues/Dynamics

J.'s parents provided their perspective on J.'s previous functioning as well as current family issues.

J.'s parents noted changes in his behavior that began last summer, in particular, that J. had a new group of friends and was out every night. This behavior continued during the school year. J.'s parents were upset about truancy and failing grades.

It was unclear at exactly what point his parents became aware of his substance abuse. They note that he depleted his $700 bank account, stole his mother's jewelry and pawned it, and sold his dirtbike as well. At this point, his parents felt he was out of control and insisted on treatment.

J.'s mother has been more directly in conflict with J. than his father as Mr. S. works a night shift and was out of the house when a lot of the arguments took place.

Mr. and Mrs. S. have been married 28 years and denied any current marital problems. They stated that Mr. S. had had a "drinking problem" that had caused considerable conflict but 5 years ago Mr. S. went for counseling and now drinks a lot less. They do not see Mr. S.'s drinking as a problem. They express some concern about their older son "who drinks," but they were vague about whether or not this was a problem. J.'s parents are willing to be involved in his treatment.

Mental Status Examination

J. presents as a tall, very thin, white male appearing his stated age of 16. He was dressed neatly in an age-appropriate fashion in blue jeans and a T-shirt. His posture was relaxed, and there was no evidence of rigidity or tension. His facial expression was mobile and mood congruent. His motor activity was normal, and there was no evidence of restlessness, dystonic reactions, or repetitive movements. Tremors were not noted. His mood was calm and somewhat dysphoric, although his affect was appropriate to thought content. His affect was also flat and somewhat constricted. His speech was in a normal tone and clear. There was no evidence of impediments or guardedness. He verbalized freely with no evidence of pressure. His thought content was logical and concrete. There was no evidence of obsessions, compulsions, ruminations, or phobias. Depersonalization and derealization were denied. Ideas of reference, persecution, or influence were denied. Delusional thinking was not evident at the time of the interview and First Rank Schneiderian Symptoms were also not present during the interview. Hallucinations, both auditory and visual, were denied. Substance-related flashbacks were denied. Homicidal ideation as well as suicidal ideating was denied at the time of the interview.

On formal mental status examination, J. was oriented in all three spheres. His fund of knowledge was appropriate to his educational level. His digit span was 4 forward and 1 in reverse. His serial 7s and 3s were calculated rapidly and accurately. His memory appeared to be intact, and there was no impairment of recent and remote memory. His intelligence appeared to be above average and his judgment appropriate. His insight appeared to be poorly developed. When asked what his three wishes would be, he replied, "to have a lot of money, a nice house, and a good family." When asked what one thing he would change about himself, he replied "I wish I were shorter." When asked what one animal he could be if he could be, he replied "an eagle." When asked where he sees himself in 5 years, he replied "in California racing dirtbikes." Patient abstracted the similarities and proverbs most concretely.

Admitting Diagnosis

- Axis I   Mixed substance abuse (cocaine, cannabis)
- Axis II   None
- Axis III   None

Physical and Neurological Examination

Physical examination revealed a height of 5'9½", weight of 127 lb, blood pressure 102/78, temperature 97.8, pulse 76, respiration 20. The general physical examination was unremarkable, including normal HEENT exam, no evidence of thyroid megaly, normal cardiovascular and pulmonary exam, and a normal abdominal exam. The neurological examination revealed intact cranial nerves, no focal neurological signs, normal sensorimotor function, and reflexes were symmetrical and normal active, as well as a normal gait and coordination. Impression was a normal neurological examination.

Laboratory Findings

On admission, laboratory test revealed a normal CBC with differential; ESR, RPR, RPR, SMA 22, urinalysis, chest X ray, and EKG, and B-12 and folate level were all WNL. A comprehensive drug screen of the urine was negative for the presence of any drugs. A sleep-deprived EEG with NP leads was normal, and a T & B cell enumeration was WNL. On transfer to the adolescent treatment unit, a drug screen also was negative for any drugs.

Psychological Testing

Psychological testing was not on the chart.

Consultations

None

Interim Diagnosis

- Axis I   Cannabis abuse, continuous alcohol abuse, episodic parent–child problem, conduct disorder, socialized, non-aggressive
- Axis II   Deferred
- Axis III   Deferred

Initial Formulation

J. presents with cannabis abuse, characterized by the daily use of cannabis since age 14 up to ⅛ an ounce per week.

There is also evidence of alcohol abuse episodic characterized by the use of alcohol on a biweekly basis. There is also a conduct disorder characterized by J.'s history of stealing, vandalism as reported by parents, truancy from school, and some selling drugs to get drugs.

Although both J. and his parents report no difficulty in the family functioning, J. reports having a conflictual relationship with his mother that contributes to a parent/child problem. Also, his father's reported drinking as well as brother's reported alcohol use may significantly contribute to this difficulty. Family and group therapy will be most helpful in dealing with this young adolescent with a drug problem.

Treatment Plan Goals and Objectives

1. Accepting the powerlessness and unmanageability over chemicals and subsequent consequences.
2. Relating the disease concept to his life.
3. Accepting and turning his life over to a higher power.
4. Taking a moral inventory of his life and sharing this in a self-disclosure to a clergyperson.
5. Building his self-esteem and assertiveness skills by having one-to-one sessions with other peers and staff, completing self-esteem assignments, requesting and accepting positive feedback from other peers and staff, sharing personal assets with other peers and staff, and being a group leader.
6. Getting in touch with emotions by sharing feelings with others in group and in one-to-one sessions.
7. Developing appropriate communication and behavior with family members by participating in family week, sharing gratitudes and resentments with family members, and honestly sharing feelings.
8. Developing a supportive environment for aftercare by discussing, interviewing, and subsequent placement in an appropriate aftercare program.

Counselors' Course in Hospital

Drug Treatment. Patient was transferred from an evaluation unit to the treatment unit on May 22, 1986. Patient was initially compliant and appeared willing to become involved in the treatment program. He was able to state that he used chemicals but denied having any problem with them. He seemed to have little understanding or willingness to look at the disease concept and how this related to him. Patient presented assignments toward his acceptance of Step I on four separate occasions and was turned down by the community each time.

Patient acted compliant at times to avoid confrontation. He also used silence, a sense of humor and blame as manipulation to keep the focus off of him. At other times, patient would test limits and would usually have difficulty in accepting the consequences of his behavior. Patient's parents came to Fair Oaks Hospital for family intervention on May 27, 1986. Patient's mother expressed feelings of anger and sadness over his lying and stealing. Patient's father agreed with mother's feedback. Patient submitted two 72-hour notices on May 29, 1986 and on June 10, 1986 at which time his parents supported continued treatment and he rescinded his 72-hour notices.

J. participated in family week from June 23–June 27, 1986 while on Status O. Patient's parents attended all week, patient's brother, age 20, and sister, age 26, each attended one day. J. expressed some feelings of guilt over hurting family members but remained in denial over the seriousness of his drug problem. He expressed a desire to stop using chemicals without the help of treatment as his brother had apparently done. Patient's mother expressed many sad and angry feelings toward patient's past drug-related behavior and present unwillingness to change, yet she would act like a caretaker and protect patient at times. Patient's mother seemed very enmeshed with patient and would often share his feelings.

Patient's father seemed better able to detach from patient and appeared in denial over his own self-admitted alcoholism. J.'s father appeared nervous throughout family week and shared very little with the group. His brother appeared able to detach from J. but seemed threatened when his own drug use was questioned. Patient's sister expressed great feelings of sadness about J. needing treatment but seemed to be the family member most comfortable with the patient's having a disease.

Patient made no progress in treatment after family week. Patients were called in to a meeting at Fair Oaks Hospital on June 22, 1986, to discuss plans for transferring patient to long-term treatment. Patient's mother showed much resistance to this suggestion at first and attempted to keep the patient in inpatient treatment at Fair Oaks Hospital. Once patient's mother fully understood the recommendation for long-term treatment, she became willing to transfer the patient. Patient's father appeared much more willing to transfer the patient than did his mother. When patient's mother and staff informed the patient of his upcoming transfer, he became angry and tried to coerce his mother into taking him home. J. spent his last week of treatment sharing feelings of sadness, anger, and fear over the transfer but continued to remain in denial over his disease.

Course in Hospital

Medical. Optimal health was maintained throughout the hospitalization. Patient was treated for a mild case of acne with Cleocin T daily, and there were no other medical problems.

Psychiatric. During the evaluation phase, patient and family were cooperative with treatment, though at one point patient requested a 72-hour discharge but retracted when resistance to treatment was worked through. Initially in the treatment program, patient displayed some shyness in talking with the group and in relating to peers. There was initial anger directed at his mother for "dumping me here." There were mild paranoid fears about being brain washed and trapped in treatment with fear that something would happen to him. He put in a 72-hour notice after 1 week, but when his parents came in to discuss this, he retracted it and seemed ready for treatment. However, over the next several weeks, patient remained resistant to treatment and oppositional when confronted in group and in individual therapy. Characteristics of the passive/aggressive personality disorder were present with resistance to demands for adequate performance, procrastination, stubbornness that appeared to be a lifelong pattern. Multiple attempts for a change in treatment were done to break through the resistance, but these met with little success, as he seemed adamant about continued drug use. This denial persisted throughout family week as evidence continued to suggest that long-term treatment would be necessary. Throughout the hospitalization, there was no evidence of psychotic signs or evidence of major depression. It was clear that maximum therapeutic benefit had been obtained from this program. Patient received no trial of psychotropic medication.

Condition upon Discharge

Medical. Patient was discharged in good health and was on no medications.

Psychiatric. Upon discharge, patient was not suicidal, depressed, or homicidal. He showed minimal progress toward treatment of his chemical dependency and of his personality disorder. Patient was discharged on no psychotropic medications.

Recommendations and Disposition

1. Referred to Golden Valley Treatment Center for continued treatment for chemical dependency.
2. Possible referral to a halfway house upon discharge from Golden Valley.
3. Upon completion of inpatient treatment, patient to attend CLEAN Teens Outpatient Program at Fair Oaks Hospital.
4. Patient to have regular attendance at a 12-step, self-help recovery program.
5. Patient's parents attend weekly parents support group with Judy Tufaro at Fair Oaks Hospital.
6. Family members to have regular attendance in a 12-step, self-help recovery program.

Final Diagnosis

- Axis I   Cannabis abuse, continuous alcohol abuse, episodic conduct disorder, socialized, nonaggressive parent–child problem
- Axis II   Passive–aggressive personality disorder
- Axis III   None

Case 3: A.

This was an emergency, voluntary admission for this 17-year-old Asian, single male. This is his first Fair Oaks admission and first psychiatric hospitalization. A. lives with his family of origin that includes his parents and two siblings. His mother S., age 37, is a nurse. His father C., age 44, is a laboratory analyst. Sister S., age 16, is a junior in high school. Brother J., age 9, is entering the fifth grade. A. has been in the eleventh grade, having been suspended 3 weeks before school closed. He is currently unemployed, having worked part-time as a busboy. Family religion is Catholic.

Chief Complaint

"Drug abuse."

History of the Present Illness

In a withholding manner, A. described increasing difficulty at school and with his mother over the past year. He related being suspended from school for the last 3 weeks of the term for truancy, cutting classes he did not like. He described failing grades in all subjects, compared to his past record of maintaining B's and C's with scattered D's.

Concurrent with school problems has been an increase in arguments with his mother with physical fighting. He reported fights would begin when he refused to comply with her request, for example, to clean the bathroom. A. said his mother would throw things, and he punched her at times to protect himself. He stated father has intervened on A.'s behalf. A. also described temper outbursts where he would hit walls. He reported living with an aunt in Florida last summer to avoid confrontations with mother. He returned to New Jersey at mother's request in the fall of 1985.

A. reported substance abuse began at age 12 with daily use of marijuana. He also has used alcohol up to an eight-pack of beer or hard liquor one to two times per week in order to potentiate the effects of marijuana and other substances. He has experimented with PCP (one time), hallucinogens for 1 week, codeine, cocaine, amphetamines, and Valium. He reported obtaining drugs with money he acquires through employment. He has worked as a busboy and waiter. He tends to terminate employment when he becomes dissatisfied with the work situation, for example, being assigned to weekend hours. Legal problems were denied, although A. admitted to an occasional involvement in providing drugs for friends. A. stated parents became aware of his drug use over the past year.

Although depressive symptoms were denied, mood appeared sad, and A. appeared to have low motivation and mild psychomotor retardation. He stated that, although mother tried to discipline him, he defies her attempts by "not listening."

A. related occasional dating, although he stated he prefers not going out with one person for too long.

Parents reported that A. has demonstrated discipline problems throughout school. He had difficulty with sitting still, although mother denied hyperactivity. He frequently engaged in fights at times involving the school principal. His fourth-grade teacher reported to parents that A. had behavioral problems in the classroom with "no self-control and does not follow directions." She also noted A. "does not respect property of others." Parents noted when A. liked the teacher, he performed better. With the family move, A. entered a Catholic school in the middle of fifth grade. Around the same time, he began cursing, and the school thought his use of curse words and his sexual interest were inappropriate. Although he would attempt extracurricular activities, he usually dropped out, not finishing a task. A. was frequently teased, and, in the sixth grade, rumors were spread that A. and another classmate had engaged in sodomy. The blame was placed on A. by the school, and grades dropped from A's and B's to C's.

Family visited the Philippines that year, and A. was introduced to smoking marijuana by a cousin. Parents reported in the eighth grade problems increased. Conferences at school indicated A. was not functioning to his potential. He tended to cut classes and not finish his homework. Mother noted A. was frightened around girls. Grades dipped further to C's and D's. Similar problems continued in eighth and ninth grades. In the ninth grade, he failed two classes and needed to attend summer school. He had engaged in several fistfights at school and was suspended for cutting classes. Cutting school continued in the tenth grade, and A. tends to hide letters from school to parents. He was suspended approximately four times during that year. He was picked up by the police for loitering with other adolescents, but no charges were pressed. It was during that year that the parents found A. inebriated, and his father noticed A. had been putting water in his Scotch. Fighting at home increased, and parents reported punishment was ineffective. Mother stated she sometimes did not follow through with threats. Parents recalled A. had frequent changes of friends and spent most of his time out of the home.

Parents reported A. has complained a lot to their family doctor about having sweaty palms.

Parents confirm A.'s living with an aunt in Florida, returning home after 1 month. Mother agreed that her relatives side with A. but viewed A.'s return as his need for peers. A. stated he did not use drugs the month he was in Florida. Parents described two runaway attempts to friends' houses lasting for 3 days.

Throughout this past year, there has been increased fighting within the family, parents state. Parents noted A. has been more explosive and cannot take criticism. He has been observed to hit the bed and has made two holes in the walls. Cutting and decreased grades have continued. A. has been verbally abusive to mother and has begun physical fighting with father.

Parents noted dysphoric mood and increase in sleeping. They state he cries easily when upset. Although A. has stated to them that he could not hurt himself, he did try at age 15 and has banged his head on walls and fights.

Past Psychiatric History

A. was seen for an evaluation at AADT. He was evaluated as chemically dependent. Parents thought that inpatient treatment would be more effective for A. and agreed to this Fair Oaks Hospital admission.

A. started his marijuana use, preferring hashish, at age 12 in the Philippines. He reported smoking marijuana all day, everyday. He has used cocaine frequently over the last year. Amphetamines have also been used infrequently since the ninth grade with no effects. He began using alcohol in the fifth grade with current use of a eight-pack of beer several times a week since the ninth grade.

Medical History

A. denied having had any medical problems. Circumcision was performed at age 8. Serious illnesses, high prolonged fevers, accidents, headaches, head injuries, seizures, speech difficulties, hearing difficulties, vision difficulties, and allergies were denied. He smokes two to three packs of cigarettes in a week.

Family Medical and Psychiatric History

Paternal uncle had a heart attack. Paternal grandmother has been treated for depression with antidepressants. Paternal grandfather died in World War II from dysentery. Several cousins have history of substance abuse.

Psychosocial and Developmental History

A. is the oldest of three children born to middle-class parents from the Philippines. He was born in the Philippines and remained there until age 3½ with his maternal grandmother. Parents came to the United States when A. was 6 months old. Mother reported that, as an infant, A. had been affectionate, warm, and loving. She weaned him at 6 months before she left for the United States. She believed A. was spoiled by her mother. Mother reported A. had a difficult adjustment to living with his parents at age 3½. By that time, his sister was born. A. described relationships with siblings as unproblematic. He stated parents get along with each other. He identified mother as the disciplinarian with "a temper." He stated father "does not impose" limits.

A. is the product of a pregnancy characterized by borderline anemia. Labor and delivery were uneventful. Birth weight was 5 lb, 6 oz. The neonatal period was within normal limits. Developmental milestones were as follows: held head up at 5 months, sat without help at 8 months, stood holding on at 10 months, rode a tricycle at 2½ years, tied shoes at 4 years, fed self at 3 years, dressed self at 3½ years, achieved toilet training at 3½ years. Language development was not recorded by mother. She stated at age 3½ A. quickly learned English upon coming to the United States. Childhood behavior was characterized by intermittent clumsiness, talking too much or too loudly, getting into things, being unable to tolerate delay, impulsiveness, inability to accept correction, fighting, unresponsiveness to discipline, not completing projects, short attention span, daydreaming, not following directions, lying, feeling left out, stealing, vandalism, demanding attention and affection, not working up to ability, and becoming easily frustrated. Difficulty with fine or gross motor skills, right–left discrimination difficulty, and difficulty learning to read were denied.

A. began public school with kindergarten and did well

in spite of attention-seeking behavior. Academically, he achieved A's, but there was a discipline problem, and, although mother denied hyperactivity, teachers complained A. had difficulty sitting still in school. Teachers reported A. took things from other children. Mother reported A. was frequently teased about being different from other children. She noted many cultural clashes. In the fourth grade, teachers stated A. was a behavioral problem in the classroom, not following directions and not respecting other peoples' property. When the family moved in the fourth grade, A. was transferred to a Catholic school that was another large adjustment for him. In the fifth grade, he began cursing, and teachers in the Catholic school noted unusual sexual interest. He frequently used curse words. Although he would involve himself in group activities, he generally dropped out. He returned to the public school in the middle of the year as the family moved again. In the sixth grade, the public school noted sexual preoccupation. At that time, grades began dropping to B's and C's. Junior high school and high school history were delineated in history of the present illness.

A. reported setting small fires once or twice. He also reported one time sitting on his cat whom he placed under a bean chair. He reported frequent school truancy. He denied vandalism and stealing, although his parents reported a history of this. He ran away for 3 days in 1985 to a friend's home. At times when he comes home after curfew, he stated his parents would lock the door and he would be required to spend the night at a friend's. He reported engaging in several physical fights at school with school suspensions. Difficulties with the police were denied.

A. reported being sexually active. He stated he has had girlfriends on occasion; however, he prefers not dating one person. Parents stated A. was anxious around girls. They reported his having the same friends since moving to the community at age 9. Parents confirmed A. having a close buddy during his childhood. He reported enjoying music, particularly playing jazz on the guitar. Up until ninth grade, he had played baseball and participated in track. He stated he was not good at these sports. He denied a vocational interest.

As stated previously, A. has worked as a busboy and waiter for several months at a time. He quits work when the situation becomes unsatisfactory, for example, when assigned to weekend hours.

Military history was denied.

Description of Current Family Issues/Dynamics

A.'s parents were seen for an interview. They see A.'s main problems as alcohol and drug abuse as well as behavioral problems. A. has a history of runaways (at friends' houses) and one time of being "kicked out" (2 days over a weekend). Parents admit they are out of control and that there has been a rise in family aggressiveness and fighting. A.'s grades dropped, and eventually he was kicked out of school for lateness and truancy (6/16/86).

Parents say that, although their marriage is not perfect and is even a volatile one, they do well, and there is not a threat of divorce. They believe A. feels unloved by them. Mother says she does have ambivalent feelings about A. and expects "perfection" from him. However, on the other hand, she admits she was often lax in keeping punishments and that she feels much guilt toward A. She harkens back to his early childhood when, because of immigration laws, she had to leave A. with his grandparents in the Philippines. She says things have not been right between the two since then and worries about this. She says she is much stressed at this point and will seek immediate help from a social worker at her work for "stress."

Mother does not drink. Father admits to occasional drinking but denies alcoholism.

Parents say A. has many friends, but they change rapidly. He has much anxiety ("sweaty palms") with girls and has not dated. Parents say some of A.'s fighting has been associated with racial slurs and comments made to him at school.

There is no current suicidality, but A. "tried something" at age 15. They say he sleeps too much and though he tries to keep himself from crying, he occasionally does.

Younger brother and older sister are said to be fine but miss A. in the house. A. is said to be especially close to his younger brother, who looks up to him. Both parents are willing to be involved in treatment.

Mental Status Examination

A. presented as a neatly dressed male appearing his stated age of 17. He appeared tense, assuming an erect position. Facial expression was fixed and congruent with his dysphoric mood. A. remained seated throughout the interview, and eye contact was established and intermittently maintained. A. appeared thin. Speech was soft, clear, and guarded, and underproductive without impediments noted. Thoughts were logical, abstract, and coherent. A. reported physically fighting with mother and peers. Hallucinations, delusions, déjà vu experiences, hypnopompic phenomenon, derealization, depersonalization, compulsions, phobias, and suicidal ideation were denied. Parents reported a past suicide attempt at age 15.

On formal testing, A. was oriented in three spheres. Fund of knowledge was fair. Remote and recent memory appeared unimpaired. Serial 7s were performed accurately and rapidly as were serial 3s. Digit span forward was 7 and 4 in reverse. Judgment responses were appropriate. Similarities and proverbs were abstracted adequately. Insight was poorly developed. A.'s three wishes were "fame, fortune, and happiness." When asked what he could change in himself, he stated "nothing—there is nothing wrong with me." He would like to be an "eagle because I want to fly." In 5 years, he stated that "I don't know what I'll be. On the top of the world."

Admitting Diagnosis

- Axis I   Conduct disorder, mixed substance abuse
- Axis II   Not established
- Axis III Not established

Physical and Neurological Examination

Physical exam revealed a height of 5'4", weight 115 lb, blood pressure 120/80, temperature 98, pulse 72. Examination was remarkable for having large but not inflamed tonsils and moderate facial acne. Remainder of the exam was unremarkable including a normal HEENT exam, nonpalpable thyroid, normal cardiovascular and pulmonary exam, and a normal abdominal exam. Neurological exam showed intact cranial nerves, no focal neurological signs; reflexes were symmetrical and hyperactive. There was a normal gait and coordination.

Laboratory Findings

Admission testing revealed a normal RPR, ESR, urinalysis, and CBC with differential. An SMA C 23 was normal except for increased LDH of 258 IU/L and increased triglycerides of 219 MG/DL. Comprehensive hepatitis evaluation was fully nonreactive. The comprehensive drug screen of the urine on admission was positive only for cannabinoids, and a serum THC at the same time was negative. A sleep-deprived EEG was done on 7/11/86 and was negative. A dexamethasone suppression test revealed normal suppression and no evidence of biological depression. A thyroid evaluation was normal except for a slightly elevated T3 uptake of 36.5% and a slightly elevated delta TSH of 15.7 UIU/ML. Several adolescent drug screens during admission were all negative.

Psychological Testing

The WAIS-R revealed a Verbal IQ of 109, Performance IQ of 102, and a Full Scale IQ of 106. WRAT-R testing revealed a reading level of 86%, spelling of 84%, and arithmetic of 45%. The test results indicated relatively preserved cognitive and intellectual functioning. Projective testing revealed an adolescent experiencing a conduct disorder with depressed mood. The latter falls within the context of a developing personality disorder with oppositional and impulsive traits. There were no signs of structural disorganization such as schizophrenia, psychosis, or even borderline pathology. There was no evidence of a breakdown on reality testing. He tended to react to situations in an emotionally detached and effectively flat manner. There was some sense that he felt different than others and did not fit in as well as revealing inner feelings of frustration and compensates for such feelings by trying to let the world know that he is some sort of strong force to be dealt with. Impression was conduct disorder with depressed mood and developing personality disorder with oppositional and impulsive traits.

Consultations

On 8/28/86, patient was seen by Dr. Becher of ENT to evaluate right ear pain. Impression: possible temporal mandibular joint problem, rule out impacted wisdom teeth. Recommendations were to see a dentist if needed.

Interim Diagnosis

- Axis I   Cannabis dependence, continuous alcohol abuse, continuous mixed substance abuse, episodic conduct disorder, undersocialized, nonaggressive, attention deficit disorder without hyperactivity, R/O major depressive disorder
- Axis II   Deferred
- Axis III   None known
- Axis IV   Severity of psychosocial stressors: deteriorating school grades, repeated suspension: 5—severe
- Axis V   Highest level of adaptive functioning this past year: 5—poor

Formulation

A. presents with a history of cannabis dependence and alcohol abuse. He has experimented with a variety of substances including cocaine, Valium, and hallucinogens. The onset of substance abuse at age 12 is concurrent with conduct disorder symptoms, undersocialized and generally nonaggressive except toward mother and occasionally peers. A. tends to have disregard for others' property and general rules. There is long-standing evidence for attention deficit disorder including short attention span, unresponsiveness to discipline, and not completing projects. In addition, there is a possibility that a depressive disorder may coexist with conduct and interest in substance abuse. Parents reported A. has a history of oversleeping, decreased appetite, and lack of motivation. Although he denies dysphoric mood, his appearance is quite dysphoric, and one is struck by A.'s feelings of hopelessness regarding the direction of his life. He conceals these feelings by stating, "there's nothing wrong with me." What his quiet, withdrawn behavior may be related to is a fear that becoming in touch with feelings will be experienced by him as intolerable. There is much conflict between A. and mother specifically, complicated by father's passivity.

Treatment Plan

Goals and objectives:

1. Accepting the powerlessness and unmanageability over chemicals and subsequent consequences.
2. Relating the disease concept to his life.
3. Accepting and turning his life over to a higher power.
4. Taking a moral inventory of his life and sharing this in a self-disclosure to a clergyperson.
5. Building his self-esteem and assertiveness skills by having one-to-one sessions with peers and staff, completing self-esteem assignments, requesting and accepting positive feedback from other peers and staff, and being a group leader.
6. Getting in touch with emotions by sharing feelings with others in group and in one-to-one sessions.
7. Developing appropriate communication and behavior with family members by participating in family week, sharing gratitudes and resentments with family members, and honestly sharing feelings.
8. Developing a supportive environment for aftercare by discussing, interviewing, and subsequent placement in an appropriate aftercare program.

Counselor's Discharge Summary

Patient was transferred from an evaluation unit to the Adolescent Center for Chemical Education, Prevention, and Treatment (ACCEPT) unit on 7/15/86. Patient initially appeared angry and was noncompliant with unit rules. He admitted he had a problem with chemicals but did not want to be in this treatment unit.

Patient had family intervention with his parents on 7/18/86. Patient's mother shared her anger at patient's chemical behavior and his disrespect of his parents. Patient's father shared the same without mother's display of emotion. Patient appeared guilty about hurting his family but enraged over something he was unable to confront his parents with.

Patient remained angry and noncompliant after his intervention. He isolated and appeared very distrustful. Patient put in 72-hour notice on 7/20/86 at 3 P.M. and rescinded it at 8 P.M. He was confronted by the community on acting superior, trying to be perfect, and avoiding feeling by smiling and laughing. On 7/25/86, patient asked the group for help and shared sadness about being in treatment and having the disease.

A family session with the patient and his parents was held on 7/29/86. Patient confronted his parents on locking him out of the house and hitting him. Patient's mother attempted to justify her actions and focused on patient's disrespect of her. Both patient and mother appeared angry and defensive. Patient's father appeared distant and avoided getting involved. Patient shared his angry feelings with his peers and his sadness over not feeling his parents' love. Although it appeared patient was sharing on a feeling level, patient remained noncompliant with unit rules and was placed on dead time (unit restrictions) on 8/4/86.

He became much less defensive within 24 hours and was taken off dead time on 8/6/86. Patient appeared to understand the disease concept and was supported by the community on 8/6/86 for having taken Step I.

Patient participated in family week from 8/18/86 to 8/22/86 as a Status 1 along with his parents, brother, and sister. Patient shared his anger and loneliness about parents' physical abuse, their high expectations, not feeling their love, and for them bringing him to this country at age 4 and taking him away from his grandparents. Patient's mother appeared guilty, angry, defensive, and unable to listen to feedback from other group members. Patient's father and siblings appeared passive and emotionally uninvolved. Parents encouraged to attend 12-step self-help recovery meetings in the community.

Patient's allegations of physical abuse were reported to the New Jersey Division of Youth and Family Services on 8/19/86. A representative of Youth and Family Services visited/interviewed the patient at this facility on 8/20/86.

Patient appeared more trustful and less defensive as he worked in family week and toward Status 2. He spoke about his low self-esteem and appeared to grasp the concept of a higher power. Patient was supported by the community on 8/23/86 for having taken Step II.

Patient soon became fearful of recovery and appeared very uncomfortable with his new healthy image. He became defensive, obnoxious, and less trustful. His status again was dropped back to 1 on 9/8/86. Patient appeared to be angry at himself and pushed himself to get more involved again. He shared about being attracted to older women as a replacement for not feeling loved by his mother. He was supported by the community on 9/13/86 for having taken Step II once again.

Patient focused on his feelings of inferiority and resentments against his family as he worked toward Status 3. He shared about being picked on as a child because of his height and nationality. He shared guilt and embarrassment over a homosexual experience. He worked on his resentments toward his parents several times but seemed unwilling to let go of them. For this, he was not supported for Status 3 on both 10/2/86 and 10/8/86 and was placed on dead time (unit restrictions) on 10/8/86. Patient appeared to work through some of his resentments by himself and was taken off dead time on 10/10/86. He shared his sadness over not being able to change his parents and felt empty inside. Patient was supported by the community on 10/18/86 for having taken Step III.

A family meeting was held without the patient on 10/10/86. Parents appeared resistive to changing their behavior and so a halfway house was recommended for the patient. They seemed somewhat agreeable to this, so patient and mother had an interview at Cedar House on 10/28/86. Patient was accepted as long as financial arrangement could be made.

Patient became very confrontive and a positive role model his last weeks in treatment. He related to many COA issues and spoke about the possibility of his father being alcoholic. (Father was encouraged to get assessed for his drinking pattern but refused.) Patient also dealt with his infatuation toward some female staff members and how his fantasies prevented him from getting close to them. Patient was supported by the community on 11/10/86 for his Status 4 after working on his issue of inferiority. Patient was discharged on 11/17/86 to Cedar House.

Course in Hospital

Medical. During the evaluation period, patient showed no signs of specific drug withdrawal. He maintained general good health throughout the hospitalization. He was treated for his moderate acne with Cleocin with good results. He was evaluated for right ear pain (see preceding section, *Consultations.* He otherwise participated in our exercise program without problems.

Psychiatric. During the evaluation period, patient was noted to have a difficult time verbalizing thoughts and feelings, tended to withdraw by playing his guitar or reading. He had begun to verbalize his dysphoria but tended to minimize problems in school and with parents. On transfer to the treatment unit, he showed significant guardedness and was reluctant to interact with other peers. He clearly stated that "I don't like people prying into me." He had significant issues regarding his parents leaving him with other family members in the Philippines at the age of 4 and suffered humiliation and abuse by his mother in the past. This was reported to the Division for Youth and Family Services who have followed the case. This guardedness was extremely severe and satisfied criteria for paranoid personality disorder. Embarrassment was the major difficulty throughout all of his treatment both on individual level and in group sessions. He began to be able to verbalize his feelings and was never expressing them out of control in a physical way. As he began to get in touch with the humiliation, he expressed wishes to die, was placed on suicidal precautions, but was able to work this through with no attempts. As these issues were dealt with, his mood became brighter and his affect became broader. The major issue throughout treatment was that of abandonment by his mother in the Philippines; however, much of his reactions were distortions of parental decisions. Family week was a significant breakthrough in the relationship with his parents, especially with his father. During the hospitalization, he intermittently showed episodes of depression; however, none were severe enough to warrant the use of antidepressants and appeared to be situational and were worked through in therapy sessions. As he began to improve, there was significant fear of being better with sabotaging of his own treatment; he had a difficulty in giving up past nonadaptive behaviors. Part of this had to do with a grandiosity and covering feelings of severe inferiority. There, arrogant defenses were used to withdraw from the community. He had fears that knowledge of certain parental activities would break up the family as if they were not able to handle this information. Much of his feelings of inferiority focused around sexual incidents at the age of 8 or 9 that were discussed and focused on, issues of rejection and humiliation. There were some identity issues as to whether he was gay, but these covered up deeper issues, feelings of weakness in general, and issues of intimacy. As he approached the termination phase of his treatment, he became a strong role model for the whole community with a wide range of affect, minimal defensiveness, and he worked well with staff and peers. A major focus of this period was to deal with issues of abandonment as he reexperienced some of the same feelings of the abandonment as well as memories from the age of 4 when he had been left in the Philippines. At this time he was able to look at them, evaluate, and change his behaviors accordingly. There was an extremely deep-seated sense of loneliness and isolation as well as differentness for which he used various people and drugs to distract and to become dependent upon. Plans were made for transfer to a halfway house to consolidate the gains that had been achieved during treatment. At no time during the hospitalization were psychotropic medications used.

Condition on Discharge

Medical. Patient was discharged in good health with weight 129 lb, height 5′6″, blood pressure 130/60, pulse 80. He had no unresolved medical problems and was discharged on no medications.

Psychiatric. Patient showed significant gains in his substance abuse problem, conduct disorder, parent/child problem, and personality disorder. Upon discharge, he was not depressed, suicidal, or homicidal. He needed continued treatment for his personality disorder and conduct disorder as well as for the parent/child problem. He was discharged on no psychotropic medications.

Recommendations and Disposition

1. Patient transferred to Cedar House, Bridgewater, New Jersey, for halfway house treatment with a focus on these issues:
   a. Integrating himself into the community and gradually back to home.
   b. Feelings of inferiority masked by superior behavior.
   c. Difficulty in forming healthy relationships with females.
   d. Letting his parents recovery and participation in treatment influence his motivation for recovery.
2. Patient to have regular attendance in a 12-step self-help recovery program.
3. Patient and parents to have weekly family therapy sessions through Catholic Charities in Bridgewater, New Jersey.
4. Parents to have regular attendance in a 12-step self-help recovery program for families.

Final Diagnosis

- Axis I   Mixed substance abuse, continuous cannabis dependence, continuous alcohol abuse, continuous conduct disorder, undersocialized, nonaggressive, attention deficit disorder, parent–child problem
- Axis II   Paranoid personality disorder
- Axis III   None

Case 4: A.

This was a voluntary, emergency admission for this 19-year-old, white, single male. This is his first psychiatric hospitalization and first Fair Oaks hospital admission. He resides in a private residence with his family: natural mother, age 49, who works as a full-time realtor, and natural father, age 53, who is a manager for an insurance company. Family religious affiliation is Protestant, and ethnic identification includes German and Irish. A. is currently in the twelfth grade. Prior to admission, he was working up to 15 hours per week for landscaping companies. Child Study Team Evaluation was completed during grade school and high school; according to parents, A. was classified *Perceptually Impaired*. A. has two natural brothers, ages 24 and 23, a full-time veterinarian student and a district manager for a plastics corporation, respectively.

Chief Complaint

"I'm here because of my vice-principal and my parents."

History of the Present Illness

A. traced the onset of alcohol use to the tenth grade when he was regularly attending parties and drinking at the rate of up to two beers per week. During the middle of the ninth grade, he had transferred schools because he "hated the junior high school" and his "peers were picking on him," he noted. A. reported that he failed academic course work at one school and then returned to public high school during the twelfth grade as his parents "did not want to keep paying for failing grades."

A. reported that he initiated friendships with a drug-user peer group at the beginning of the twelfth grade; he noted that his grades continued to decline from the eleventh grade when he was failing courses. He noted that, during the twelfth grade, he was late to class consistently and had multiple detentions. He was once suspended in the eleventh grade for a 3-day period for "kicking a water fountain."

A. reported that he was arrested once for breaking and entering during the eighth grade; probation lasted through 1987. He denied any current probation. Just prior to admission, A. stated that he served a 5-day suspension for marijuana usage in school. During the twelfth grade, A. noted that he stopped using marijuana for periods of time but was generally unsuccessful. He identified that his alcohol consumption had progressed to regular weekend use, up to three times per weekend.

A. stated that school authorities mandated an evaluation for drug abuse, and he attended AADT for 6 months of outpatient treatment; he noted that he first went to AADT during the eleventh grade and participated in regular urine screening. He noted that he was noncompliant with the outpatient program. On 4/26/88, A. participated in an evaluation session at Outpatient Recovery Center located at Fair Oaks Hospital, and inpatient psychiatric treatment for substance rehabilitation was recommended.

A. reported that in 1981 his maternal grandmother died. He identified weekly bouts of depression characterized by fleeting suicidal ideation and planning during the tenth grade as he "was standing on the roof of a building threatening to fall off." He also identified a history of racing thoughts. He also noted a consistent history of difficulty falling asleep.

Over the past 1-year prior to admission, A. reported abuse of the family dog as he has regularly "kicked the dog." His parents are in the process of "getting rid of the dog which was his Christmas gift," according to A.

In addition, A. has been anticipating graduation from high school and attending college thereafter. Father and A. stated that a tentative plan consisted of A. attending college out of state and living with his one natural brother; both expressed concern regarding the availability of drugs and alcohol in this environment.

Past Psychiatric History

Any past psychiatric, inpatient, or residential treatment was denied. A. reported that he participated in weekly, individual sessions with a psychoanalyst for a period of 3 months in 1987; he noted that it was recommended to parents that he "pay for property destroyed." A. also reported participation in monthly sessions between the eleventh and twelfth grades for a period of 6 months; monthly urine screens were obtained, and A. reported that his first urine screen was positive and the remaining five were negative. He also participated in an unspecified number of sessions with a school psychiatrist. A. denied any past use of psychiatric medications for any reason.

His parents reported that between the third and forth grades, A. was classified *Perceptually Impaired* as he was initially considered dyslexic. Parents reported that A. attended both regular and special education classes throughout grammar school.

A.'s history of substances experimentation was reported including the following: "hashish" (unknown amount, once only) used in the spring of 1986; cocaine (up to 10 lines, once only) used via inhalation method used at the age of 17; amphetamines (No-Dozs, up to 13 pills, at once) used in the spring of 1986 that resulted in nausea and vomiting; "rush" (up to two inhalations, once only) used during the winter of 1986; and "whippits" (up to six cartridges on two occasions and one balloon on two occasions) during the winter of 1988. Current drugs of choice have included marijuana (up to one-quarter ounce every other day), first use at the age of 16 and last used on 4/13/88, and alcohol (up to 24 beers in a 2-hour period on a weekly basis or up to eight shots per night, on a weekly basis).

Medical History

A. recalled normal childhood illnesses including chickenpox. Immunizations were reportedly up to date, whereas allergies were denied. Any incident of high, prolonged fever was also denied. He reported the occurrence of three car accidents with his own motor vehicles; one accident occurred when he "ran a red light." A history of temporal lobe, monthly headaches were reported that were typically relieved by aspirin. Any history of fractures was denied. At the age of 18, a head injury occurred during the summer of 1987 when A. was "kicked in the head," which resulted in a loss of consciousness for approximately 3 minutes, according to an eyewitness account, A. reported. This injury also resulted in a severe headache and tinnitus, although he had attended a live concert while experiencing these postconcussive symptoms. At the age of 8, A. recalled in a dream when a dog bit him on the left shoulder, which required four stitches; at the age of 6 he received stitches to his throat after an injury while playing the flute. At the age of 8, A. underwent a surgical repair for septum without complications. He denied any past history of venereal or thyroid disease, hepatitis, difficulties in speech or hearing, and color blindness. Vision difficulties have included the occurrence of left eye pain that occurs on the average of four times per year.

In regard to nutritional status, A. typically eats three meals per day, he reported. At times he experiences left jaw pain and therefore eats slowly. He described a "hardy appetite" and weighs approximately 139 pounds. He also reported that his weight tends to fluctuate between 135 and 145 pounds. At the age of 18, school authorities sent him to Smoke Enders, which he successfully completed. However, he has smoked up to five packs per day since the eighth grade; his cigarette usage has progressively increased throughout high-school years. Alcohol has been used on a regular basis since the age of 15, and A. stated that his use has varied with his mood. In addition to alcohol, marijuana was reported as his other drug of choice, used since age 16. Other medical problems have included the diagnosis of mitral valve prolapse via echocardiogram in 1/88 according to A. Characteristically, A. has reported the occurrence of sweaty palms and tingling of the legs and feet.

Family Medical and Psychiatric History

Any significant family psychiatric history was denied. Maternal grandmother is alive; she has been diagnosed with cancer and suffers from arthritis. Maternal grandfather died from a heart attack. Paternal grandparents are both deceased; grandmother died in 1981, and she suffered from arthritis, and grandfather was diagnosed with Alzheimer's disease, A. reported.

Psychosocial and Developmental History

A. is the youngest of three natural children born to parents from a upper-middle-class family. His early childhood memories are "happy ones." And he described a "great marital relationship" between his parents as a history of discord and violence was denied. He noted that his mother "cared about me" and his father "usually arrived home at 5:00 and told me to do chores." A. denied that his parents were separated or divorced. Family's religious affiliation is Protestant, and A. recalled participation in church activities during childhood.

According to parents, A. refused to go to bed when he was approximately 18 months of age. They reported excellent gross motor coordination; in addition, parents had to "place a harness on his crib so that he would not leave the house." Parents also stated that A. refused to drink milk during his infancy. Parents did not provide information regarding neonatal and birth histories or the attainment of developmental milestones.

In regard to school performance, parents noted that A. had an "excellent memory." They stated that A. was retained during the second grade and that, in general, his academic grades were poor. Between the third and fourth grades, A. was classified as *perceptually impaired*, and he was placed in special education classes. Dyslexia was considered as a possible diagnosis prior to the Child Study Team Evaluation, at that time. He was enrolled in math tutoring classes during one of his summers in grammar school. He achieved an overall C average "without doing homework" during his junior high-school years, his parents stated. He then transferred to private school, where he did fairly well, according to his parents, for the first three semesters during the ninth and tenth grades. During the last semester of the tenth grade, A. received a failing grade for biology; he was consistently late to class. During the tenth grade, parents first started to suspect drug abuse. They denied that A. was active in his community or extracurricular activities during the tenth grade. Grades began to decline and he had difficulties with his peer group, they noted. In addition, his parents noted that during the tenth grade, A. received his driving license and had six accidents in a 2-year period. Parents stated that he would either "lose control of the vehicle or fall asleep." During the eleventh grade, A. transferred to Summit Public High School; he was enrolled in a vocational school program. Parents noted that A. has always wanted to attend college. Parents reported that A. has been accepted to college, where he wants to major in the biomedical field. A. denied any past difficulties in gross or fine motor skills or right–left discrimination. He reported that he is right-hand-dominant. Difficulties in letter reversals were described since the sixth grade through the present time, but A. noted that this condition has improved. He denied any difficulties in attention span or concentration. A. confirmed that he utilized resource room during the eighth grade and attended remedial classes during the sixth and seventh grades. He noted that his best subjects have included gym and photography and his worst have been history and law. A. denied any out-of-school suspensions but noted a multitude of in-school suspensions during the eleventh and twelfth grades; he recalled a total of five for smoking, kicking a water fountain, and using marijuana. He denied any history of bizarre or habitual behaviors, enuresis, encopresis, or property destruction. He described abuse of the family dog over this past 1 year prior to admission. He also reported up to three head-banging incidences per year; he noted that 1 week prior to hospitalization, he "smashed his head" because of difficulties with a girlfriend. He described setting controlled fires in the woods with other male peers. A.'s history of stealing was also described; he reported stealing four tires at the age of 17 and stealing up to $2,000 worth of merchandise from a school, at the age of 15, resulting in a 3-year probationary period. During the fifth grade, A. recalled thinking about running away because he "did not want to take piano lessons any longer." He reported involvement in one physical fight per year, noting that he is usually provoked because peers "pick on me." One legal arrest resulted from the breaking and entering at the age of 15, which resulted in the probationary period and 25 hours of community service. A. noted that his probationary period was terminated 1½ years earlier due to "good behavior."

In regard to social relationships, A. reported that some of his current friends are drug users. He noted that his first date was in the seventh grade and his first sexual experience, which was forced by his natural brother, was at the age of 6.

He added that his first sexual experience, by choice, was at the age of 16. Parents stated that A. has maintained long-term relationships with peers. A. reported that he has enjoyed archery, model building, pool, bowling, and hackey-sack.

Parents reported that A. has held a number of odd jobs in the past. A. stated that his first job was as a busboy at a restaurant that he held for a 1-year period on a part-time basis. His second job, he stated, was as a cook, which he held for a 6-month period. His third job, which is his current employment, is part-time work through landscaping companies at a rate of up to 15 hours per week. In the future, A. noted that he would like to go to college to become a biomedical technician; to date, he has been accepted to a 2-year technical college located in Connecticut, which is located close to his brother's residence.

Military history was denied.

Legal history consisted of one arrest for breaking and entering in which A. stole $2,000 worth of merchandise from a school. He was sentenced to a 3-year probationary period and 25 hours of community service, which he has completed.

Mental Status Examination

At the time of this interview, A. appeared as a cooperative, average-looking, fair-haired young male who is dressed in a disheveled manner and resembles his stated age of 19. Posture was relaxed as he lay recumbent on the bed throughout the interview. Facial expression was mobile and mood-congruent. Motor activity was normal but somewhat restless. He fidgeted, at times, throughout the interview. Mood was calm but anxious. Affect seemed appropriate to content and demonstrated full range. He freely verbalized in a sometimes pressured fashion using a clear and normal tone of voice. Content of thoughts was logical and adequately abstract as he abstracted four out of seven similarities and three out of three proverbs. He described ideas of influence related to his reading of literature on satanism as he once felt "all-powerful." There was no evidence of obsessions, compulsions, ruminations, phobias, depersonalization, derealization, suspiciousness, ideas of reference, ideas of persecution, or delusions. Schneiderian first-rank symptoms were also denied. There was no evidence of hallucinations, hypnogogic or hypnopompic phenomenon, déjà vu and jaimais vu experience or substances-related flashbacks. He expressed homicidal ideation toward schoolteachers and one male peer who is currently at Fair Oaks Hospital for inpatient treatment. Homicidal planning included the use of a gun and a bow and arrow. Any past homicidal attempts were denied. Suicidal ideation and planning was denied, although one gesture was described at the age of 17 when he carved "kill John" onto his left arm with a razor while under the influence of alcohol. A history of hypomania and depression was denied.

Formal mental status examination found A. oriented to three spheres. Fund of knowledge was good and appropriate to his educational level. Recent and remote memory appeared intact. He calculated serial 7s slowly with errors and serial 3s rapidly and accurately. Digit span forward was 7 and reverse was 5. Judgment seemed impaired; when asked what he would do if he lost a book belonging to the library, he stated, "not worry too much." Three wishes included, "graduate high school, get out of Fair Oaks Hospital, and get my ex-girlfriend, K., back." If he could change one thing about himself, A. stated, "my age, I'd like to be older or I'd like to be a baby again." If he could be an animal, A. stated that he would like to be a pterodactyl. In 5 years from now, A. envisioned himself in the following manner: "I'll have a house, car, wife, or long-term relationship; I'll have a job and children if I'm married." He reported that his favorite movie is "Night to Remember," favorite TV show is "Family Ties" and

"Flintstones," and favorite music/rock group is "Heavy Metal/Slayer."

Formulation

A. presents with a history of behaviors compatible with attention-deficit hyperactivity disorder characterized by school problems, acting-out behaviors, and dyslexia. He was classified as *perceptually impaired* between the third and fourth grades by the Child Study Team. A low frustration tolerance is noted. The onset of alcohol use was dated to the tenth grade; A. uses alcohol at a rate of up to 24 beers per night on a weekly basis, particularly on weekends. His other drug of choice includes marijuana used since the age of 16 at the rate of up to one-quarter ounce on an every-other-day basis. He reports experimentation with "hashish," amphetamines including No-Dozs, cocaine, and inhalants including "rush" and "whippets." He was noncompliant with outpatient drug screening in which he participated for a 6-month period prior to this admission. Since the tenth grade, A.'s academic performance has declined. Parents report that he was involved in six car accidents after receiving his driver's license; A. reports three car accidents. At the age of 18, he suffered a head injury resulting in loss of consciousness. He reports that mitral valve prolapse was diagnosed via echocardiogram in 1/88. A. reported the occurrence of five suspensions between the eleventh and twelfth grades. He also reports a history of head banging. Restlessness and fidgeting have been observed during this Fair Oaks Hospital admission. He expressed homicidal ideation and plans toward schoolteachers and one male peer. Educational and vocational planning may provide a focus for future treatment during the course of this hospitalization.

Diagnostic Impression

- Axis I   Conduct disorder, solitary, aggressive, attention deficit-hyperactivity disorder, alcohol dependence, severe cannabis dependence, severe
- Axis II   R/O specific developmental disorders
- Axis III   R/O sequela to head injury with loss of consciousness
- Axis IV   Severity of psychosocial stressors: change of schools during the eleventh grade; death of paternal grandmother in 1981; arrest for breaking and entering at the age of 15 resulting in 3-year probationary period and community service; total of five suspensions during the eleventh and twelfth grades; pressure experienced by A. from parents to move out of the family home and attend college during this next academic year; anticipation of future school plans related to acceptance to 2-year vocational school in Connecticut where natural brother resides.

        Severity: 4-severe

Case 5: J.

This was a voluntary, emergency admission for the 18-year-old white male. This is J.'s first psychiatric hospitalization and first Fair Oaks Hospital admission. He resides with his family: natural mother, age 45, who works as a full-time secretary in a corporation; natural brother, age 16, who is in the tenth grade, and natural sister, age 13, who is in the eighth grade. Family religious affiliation is Protestant, and ethnic identification includes Irish, Finnish, and English. He is currently in the twelfth grade. He is employed as a waiter up to 18 hours per week and also works as a land surveyor for a family-operated business up to 8 hours per week. J. is single. Any past Child Study Team Evaluation was denied.

Chief Complaint

"I have a problem with pot and when I drink alcohol, I drink too much."

History of the Present Illness

J. traced the onset of marijuana use to freshman year of high school when he was introduced to marijuana by other freshmen in his class; he stated that he immediately "liked it" at that time. He smoked up to a ¼ joint on a monthly basis in his freshman year of high school, indicating that he enjoyed smoking alone and with friends. He was earning C grades during his freshman year, he recalled. During the ninth grade, his father was living in an apartment where he generally would stay on the weekends; he noted that his parents divorced when he was in the eighth grade.

In the tenth grade, marijuana usage increased up to twice per week; his use was generally with friends after school hours, he recalled. There was no significant change in his grades during the tenth grade, he noted.

His first use of alcohol was during the summer just prior to the tenth grade when he drank up to one standard bottle of Canadian Club whiskey and "blacked out." He was curious to discover "what it would be like to get drunk," he stated. At the time of this intoxication episode, he was with a male friend. During the summer prior to the eleventh grade, J. experimented with marijuana on one occasion; he recalled that he had a significant amount of free time during the summer months, as he was working part time.

During the eleventh grade, J. bought a car, and the first relationship with a girlfriend occurred at this time, J. reported. He began to attend parties, initially, on a weekly basis. He stated that he was using marijuana up to three times per week. He continued to consume alcohol on a weekly basis but denies "drinking and driving."

J. stated that he experimented with cocaine for the first time during the eleventh grade (spring of 1987) via a friend at his place of employment. He noted that he had used cocaine (up to 10 lines, up to 5 times total) with last use noted in 12/87. J. noted that during the end of the eleventh grade, marijuana usage increased to up to one joint, three times per week.

J. reported that he failed his first class during the eleventh grade; he recalled hating school by the spring of 1987.

After J. bought his own car, J.'s father and he had more conflict regarding the amount of time spent together. J. wanted to "party with his friends." Significantly, his father remarried in 9/87 while J. was in his junior year of high school. He recalled that his father had dated his stepmother since the beginning of his sophomore year. During the summer of 1987, J. met his current girlfriend of 10 months. He began smoking up to three joints per day, and alcohol usage increased due to socializing with his girlfriend and her friends. At the end of the summer of 1987, his girlfriend left for college. After she left, his use of marijuana increased slightly. He continued to consume alcohol mostly on weekends. During the fall of 1987, he recalled feeling "unhappy" and believed that he needed to decrease his drug usage. Therefore, he began smoking only five times per week compared to daily use. In September of 1987, J. recalled that he experimented with "mushrooms" and alcohol, mixed, while attending a concert. During September of 1987, J. recalled failing English; he had lost interest in school and generally felt "bored." He denied any involvement in school or community activities at that time. During the winter of 1987, J. was consuming alcohol at a rate of up to seven shots per night, up to twice per week. He experienced an increased level of boredom during the winter months.

In March of 1988, J. reported that he, "for the most part," stopped drinking alcohol. His marijuana usage was at the rate of up to five times per week, up to seven joints per day.

Recent psychosocial stressors have clearly included father's remarriage in 9/87 and poor relationship with stepmother.

J. reported that his current drugs of choice include marijuana (up to seven joints every day) with last use noted on 5/2/88; positive effects of marijuana have included its ability to "kill boredom," and negative effects have included lack of energy, lack of motivation, and tendency to procrastinate. Alcohol (up to seven shots of hard liquor, biweekly use, and up to seven beers on a monthly basis) has also been used to "kill boredom," and negative effects reported have included up to a total of four blackouts, up to a total of five hangovers, exacerbation of depression, decrease in level of inhibition, and lack of awareness regarding his limits.

Past Psychiatric History

Any past inpatient or residual psychiatric treatment was denied. He reported participating in up to four individual sessions with a clinical psychologist, from April through May of 1987; J. noted that the sessions addressed "conflict with his father" and added that he was "not completely honest." Various psychological tests were completed, at that time, including an MMPI that proved normal, he reported. J. stated that he also participated in an evaluation session with the Outpatient Recovery Center of FOH at which time a recommendation for inpatient psychiatric treatment for drug rehabilitation was made. J. denied any past use of psychiatric medications.

A history of drug experimentation was described. At the age of 15, J. inhaled "whippets" (up to one hit, three times total), last used at the age of 16. In 9/86, J. reported the use of hashish (up to ¼ gram, once per week) used through 12/86 that caused a decreased level of energy. Cocaine was first used in the spring of 1987 (up to 10 lines over a 7-hour period, up to 5 times total) and last used in December of 1987 via inhalation method, he recalled. "Mushrooms" were used on 9/4/87 at the rate of up to four small pieces, once only, he noted. During the winter of 1987, J. reported the use of Ritalin (up to 90 mg, three times total) that decreased his appetite, caused insomnia and muscle cramps. In April of 1987, J. noted that he used Valium (up to three tabs, up to three times total) which produced a "mellow" experience. J. added that the Ritalin was his brother's prescription and was located in the family home.

Medical History

J. reported normal childhood illnesses including a bout of chickenpox and pneumonia at the age of 6 months. He recalled 2 episodes of bronchitis during childhood. Immunizations were reportedly up to date. All allergies were denied. One episode of high, prolonged fever was recalled at the age of 5 for which an ice bath was given. At the age of 17, he described involvement in a car accident, resulting in a minor "whiplash" for which he was prescribed a muscle relaxant, Soma (dosage and frequency unknown), for a period of time. J. reported the occurrence of headaches on the average of once every 3 months; he also associated headaches with a total of five hangovers related to excessive alcohol use. Any history of fractures was denied. At the age of 12, a head injury was recalled that was related to a pool accident. During this incident, J. lost consciousness for several minutes after which he experienced a severe headache, vomiting, blurry vision, and excessive fatigue. Any history of seizure activity was denied. Medical hospitalizations have included surgical repair of hernia at the age of 6 without complications. On an outpatient basis, J. reported that a benign cyst was surgically removed from his left hand that required several stitches at the age of 15. Any history of venereal or thyroid disease, hepatitis, difficulties in speech or hearing, or color blindness was denied. A history of vision difficulties has included a condition of nearsightedness diagnosed in the eighth grade for which prescription glasses were worn; J. noted that he has worn contact lenses since the tenth grade. During the seventh grade, J. recalled a wrestling injury for which an orthopedic workup was completed; a series of prescribed back-strengthening exercises were recommended to J.

J. reported an increased appetite that was correlated with marijuana usage over the last several years; current weight is approximately 170 lb, and he denies any recent weight loss. Alcohol usage has included up to seven shots of hard liquor on a biweekly basis particularly since the eleventh grade. J. also reported a history of marijuana (up to seven joints per day), use and experimentation with various substances including cocaine, Valium, and hashish (up to ¼ gram, on a weekly basis) used over a 3-month period.

Family Medical and Psychiatric History

A significant history of alcoholism, substance abuse, depression, and thyroid disease is noted among J.'s family members. Father and J. reported that the mother has suffered from alcoholism. One maternal uncle has also suffered from alcoholism, a history of drug abuse, eccentric behavior, and has a delinquency record and a history of violent episodes. One out of two maternal aunts has also suffered from alcoholism. Maternal grandmother suffered from depression and made a suicide attempt via an overdose of Valium. Paternal grandfather had been hospitalized in the past and was treated with antipsychotics and antidepressants.

Cardiovascular disease was noted in one paternal family member; cerebrovascular disease was noted in one maternal family member. Father reported that he and paternal grandmother have suffered from thyroid disease. Diabetes is noted in one paternal aunt. Father also noted that paternal grandfather has suffered from skin cancer. Father also stated that maternal grandfather may have suffered from an alcohol problem.

Psychosocial and Developmental History

J. is the oldest of three natural children. During the eighth grade, parents separated and divorced approximately 1½ years later. J. has three stepbrothers from his father's second marriage, because his stepmother was married previously. During his childhood, he noted that his mother "would always listen; she had a drinking problem, but it never affected me." He described his father as "spending time with all of us; I learned a lot from him as he was supportive." J. described a "good marital relationship" as his parents "almost never fought." He recalled more family tension prior to their separation and stated that "my mother wanted to separate; she quit drinking." He also stated that his parents are "completely different people." In regard to relationships with his natural siblings, he stated that they get angry at one another, but issues of conflict are generally resolved. J. stated that both of his parents share custody for him and his natural siblings. In 9/87, his father remarried; his mother has remained single. In regard to current visitation plans, J. was living with his father and stepmother on weekends; due to increased conflict with his father, J. has refused to spend time with father and stepmother. He noted that both of his natural siblings continue to live with his father on weekends. Family religious affiliation is Protestant; he described a history of being active in church activities through the summer of 1987.

Mother reported that birth and neonatal history were unremarkable, although forceps were utilized and anesthesia and other medication was given at the time of delivery. Slight yellow jaundice and bruises were noted at the time of delivery. Birth weight was 7 lb, 15 oz. During infancy, mother noted that J. was colicky for approximately 1 month. She recalled that J. suffered a bout of pneumonia at the age of 6 months. She recalled the following ages of attainment for developmental skills: sat without help at 6 months; crawled at 9 months; stood at 9 months; stood holding on at 9 months; fed self at 1 year; dressed self at 2 years; stayed dry during the day and night at 2½ years; achieved bowel control at 2½ years; and spoke first word at 11 months. She stated that he named objects and put two to three words together at "a very early age." She reported that J. was left-handed during childhood. J. denied any past difficulties in gross or fine motor skills, right–left discrimination, letter reversal, or attention span. He reported some difficulty with concentration over the past 2 years and has "needed to read the same material twice since his mind tends to wander." In contrast to his mother's report, J. indicated that he is right-hand-dominant. J. further denied any history of bizarre/habitual behaviors, head banging/rocking, encopresis, or cruelty to animals. During his freshman year of high school, he and a group of friends started a dry-leaf fire and also "shot off fireworks." During "mischief night" in high school, J. reported being with a group of peers who put shaving cream on someone's property and who stole from neighbors. J. denied any past runaway incidents. He further denied any history of physical aggression or assault.

In regard to educational history, J. entered kindergarten at the age of 5; he reported achieving good grades throughout grammar school. He was placed in an advanced reading class through the third grade, he reported. During the seventh grade, J. noted that his grades began to decline, resulting in a C average during high-school years. He denied any suspensions or expulsions from school. He reported truant behavior during his senior year for a total of up to 2½ days. Mother described J.'s academic performance as progressively declining throughout his school years; in the eleventh grade, she noted that he failed geometry. She denied, however, any specific difficulties in learning. J. always attended public school. Mother denied that he was ever referred for a Child Study Team evaluation.

J. reported that it has always been easy for him to make friends; he met his best friend in kindergarten and noted that he has been able to maintain long-term relationships. He was unable to recall when his first date occurred. During his freshmen year, he noted that he engaged in his first sexual experience and has continued to remain sexually active throughout high school. Mother noted that J.'s personality was outgoing throughout all of his school years. She denied that the family was ever advised to delay entering J. into kindergarten due to immaturity. She stated that his social adjustment with peers was excellent throughout all of his school years. She denied any history of behavioral problems in the classroom. In regard to dating history, his mother noted that J. has participated in a few long-standing relationships. J. reported that he had been involved in the Key Club during his sophomore and junior years of high school. He had also been the vice president of a youth group at his church; these church activities stopped during the summer of 1987. He stated that, during his early years of high school, all of his friends were church-related contacts.

In regard to employment history, J.'s first and current job began at the age of 16; he has worked as a part-time waiter for approximately 2½ years. He has also worked for a family-operated business as a land surveyor. In regard to future career interests, J. noted that he wants to pursue further studies in psychology or business.

In regard to legal difficulties, J. reported police contact on one occasion when three of his male friends were consuming alcohol in his car. J. denied that he was drinking because he was not in the car at the time. He reported that the police returned his car keys to him and arrested his three friends.

Mental Status Examination

At the time of this interview, J. appeared as a cooperative, average, neatly groomed adolescent resembling his stated age of 18. Posture was relaxed as he sat erect in a chair throughout the interview. Facial expression was mobile and mood-congruent. Motor activity was normal. Mood was calm, and affect was somewhat constricted but appropriate to content. He freely verbalized in a clear and normal tone of voice. Content of thought was logical and adequately abstract as he abstracted six out of seven similarities and three out of three proverbs. There was no evidence of obsessions, compulsions, ruminations, depersonalization, derealization, suspiciousness, ideas of reference, ideas of persecution, ideas of influence, or delusions. An excessive fear of bridges and deep water was noted. Schneiderian first-rank symptoms were denied. All types of hallucinations, hypnagogic and hypnopompic phenonomen, jamais vu experiences and substance-related flashbacks were denied. He noted the occurrence of déjà vu experiences on a biyearly basis. Homicidal ideation in regard to a dream consisting of a "male who cheated on his wife" was described. Any homicidal plans or attempts were denied. Suicidal ideation was described as "fleeting thoughts" from 9/87 through 3/88. However, suicidal planning or attempts were denied. Any history of hypomania was denied. The present symptomatology has included a decline in academic performance since the eleventh grade, dysphoric mood, lack of energy, decline in level of interest in outside activities, difficulty concentrating, and fleeting suicidal ideation.

Formal mental status examination found J. oriented to three spheres. Fund of knowledge was appropriate to educational level. Recent and remote memory appeared intact. Serial 7s were performed accurately but slowly; serial 3s were performed rapidly and accurately. Digit span forward was 6 and reverse was 6. Social and personal judgment responses seemed inappropriate. However, insight was adequate. Three wishes included: "that there be an easy way to take care of my addiction; be with my girlfriend; and go to my graduation." If he could change one thing about himself, J. noted, "my drug addiction." If he could be an animal, J. stated, "I'd be a cat since they just hang out." In 5 years from now, J. envisioned himself in the following manner: "I'll have a job and be out of college; I'll have a lot of fun and move up at work. I'll probably lead a Yuppie life-style." He reported that his favorite movie is "The Big Chill," his favorite TV show is "Married with Children," and favorite music/rock group is "rock and roll/Rolling Stones."

Formulation

J. presents with an essentially 3-year history of substance abuse including marijuana (up to seven joints every day) and alcohol (up to seven shots of hard liquor biweekly or up to seven beers on a monthly basis). He also reports a history of experimentation with "mushrooms," "whippets," cocaine, Ritalin (brother's prescription), and Valium. In addition, J. reports the use of "hashish" from 9/86 through 12/86 at a rate of up to $\frac{1}{4}$ gram on a weekly basis. J. minimizes the effect of his natural mother's alcoholism on him or his family. Natural parents first separated when J. was in the eighth grade and

divorced approximately 1½ years later. Natural father remarried in 9/87; he relates poorly to his stepmother. Some
depressive symptomatology is described and includes the following: progressive decline in academic performance since
the seventh grade with academic failure noted in the eleventh
grade; dysphoric mood; lack of energy; anhedonia; poor concentration, and fleeting suicidal ideation. At the age of 12, J.
reports a severe head injury that resulted in a concussion
while swimming in a pool. He describes excessive fearfulness
of bridges and deep water. In 9/87, he terminated his relationship with his first girlfriend and experienced a decline in
self-esteem because he was dating two girls at the same time
about which he felt guilt. In addition, his father remarried in
9/87, and he recalled the onset of dysphoric mood at that time.
In general, he experienced a higher stress level since 9/87.

Diagnostic Impression

- Axis I   Marijuana dependence, severe alcohol de-
                pendence, moderate parent–child prob-
                lem; simple phobia (bridges), R/O de-
                pressive disorder NOS
- Axis II   Deferred
- Axis III   R/O sequela to head injury with concus-
                sion, age 12
- Axis IV   Severity of psychosocial stressors: Father
                remarried in 9/87; termination of rela-
                tionship with first girlfriend in 9/87

References

1. Schwartz RH, Hawks RL: Toward optimal laboratory use: Laboratory detection of marijuana use. *JAMA* 1985;254:788–792.
2. Gold MS, Pottash ALC, Estroff TW: Substance-induced organic

mental disorders, in Hales RE, Frances AJ (eds), *Psychiatry Update*. Washington, DC, APA Press, 1985:227–240.
3. Estroff TW, Gold MS: Psychiatric presentations of marijuana abuse. *Psychiatric Annals* 1986;16:221–224.
4. Dackis CA, Gold MS, Estroff TW: Inpatient treatment of addiction, in *APA Manual of Therapeutics*. Washington, DC, APA Press (in press).
5. Tunving K: Psychiatric effects of cannabis use. *Acta Psychiatr Scand* 1985;72:209–217.
6. Tennant FS, Groesbeck CJ: Psychiatric effects of hashish. *Arch Gen Psychiatry* 1972;27:133–136.
7. Williams RL, Karacan I: Sleep disorders diagnosis and treatment. New York, Wiley, 1978.
8. Fink M: Effects of acute and chronic inhalation of hashish, marijuana and delta-9-tetrahydrocannabinol on brain electrical activity in man: Evidence for tissue tolerance. *Ann NY Acad Sci* 1976;282:387–397.
9. Jones RT, Benzowitz N, Bachman JA: Clinical studies of cannabis tolerance and dependence. *Ann NY Acad Sci* 1976;282:221–239.
10. Miller JD et al: National survey on drug abuse: Main findings. Rockville, MD, National Institute of Drug Abuse, 1985.
11. Goodwin DW: Alcoholism and heredity. *Arch Gen Psychiatry* 1979;36:57–61.
12. Goodwin DW: Alcoholism and genetics. *Arch Gen Psychiatry* 1985;171–174.
13. Cadoret R, Garth A: Inheritance of alcoholism in adoptees. *Br J Psychiatry* 1978;132:252–288.
14. Jaffe JH: Drug and addiction abuse, in Goodman LS, Gilman AG, Rall TW, Murad F (eds), *The Pharmacological Basis of Therapeutics*. New York, Macmillan, ed 7, 1985:532–581.
15. Miller NS: A primer for the treatment process for alcohol and drug addiction. *Psychiatry Letter* 1987;5(7):30–37.
16. Miller NS, Gold MS: Marijuana (cannabis) dependence (addiction) and consequences. *J Substance Abuse* (in press).
17. Galizio M, Maisto SA: *Determinants of substance abuse*. New York, Plenum Press, 1985.
18. Harris LS, Dewey WL, Razdan RK: Cannabis: Its chemistry, pharmacology, and toxicology, in Martin WR (ed), *Drug Addiction*. Berlin, Springer-Verlag, 1977.

6

Laboratory Detection of Marijuana Use

A number of laboratory tests detect the presence of cannabinoids. The choice of test depends primarily on its purpose—whether it is to serve as a screening tool, to confirm a diagnosis of marijuana abuse in an individual patient, or to monitor the results of a patient's treatment program. The fundamental trade-off among the various techniques is low cost and/or ease-of-use versus accuracy.

Unlike blood-alcohol tests, marijuana urine-testing cannot reliably be correlated with concurrent behavioral effects, that is, a positive test result does not imply that the subject was "high" when he or she provided the sample. Because of the pharmacokinetics of cannabinoids, circulating blood levels have little to do with reported subjective effects (see Chapter 2). They do, however, correlate with motor impairment. Urinalysis establishes only that marijuana use has occurred within the several weeks preceding collection of the specimen. Salivary tests can narrow this time frame to about twelve hours, but it must be kept in mind that all of these tests provide evidence of marijuana *use*, not of intoxication. Intoxication or impairment must be established by a formal mental-status examination and a careful history.

Overview: Laboratory Testing Methods

Thin-Layer Chromatography

Thin-layer chromatography (TLC) is performed by removing the liquid portion of the urine and chemically treating the residue to separate its various chemical compounds. A dye solution sprayed on the treated sample causes color changes.

Individual drugs are identified visually on the chromatography column by their location and color. TLC can test for as many as 40 drugs from a single urine sample. The most commonly used TLC test is the TOXI-LAB (Analytical Systems, Marion Laboratories).

Although TLC is inexpensive and can identify a wide range of drugs, it is not as sensitive as other tests. Results require a subjective judgment on the part of the technician; thus, the test is subject to error, especially for borderline cases when cannabinoid levels in the urine are low. In general, drug levels of 1000–2000 ng/ml are required for positive identification—versus levels as low as 20 ng/ml for enzyme immunoassay.[1] In addition, the dyes used in TLC fade quickly, making later review of the results impossible unless a photograph is made of the test.

Immunoassay

Enzyme immunoassay (EIA) and radioimmunoassay (RIA), both of which use antibodies that attach themselves to cannabinoids in the urine, offer a rapid, low-cost method of testing. EIA may be performed in the office, but RIA must be performed in a specially licensed laboratory, because of radiolabeled antibodies.

The major drawback to immunoassays is cross-reactivity resulting in false-positive results. A number of substances, such as ibuprofen, may mimic marijuana in both EIA and RIA tests. In addition, adulterants in the urine sample such as vinegar, sodium chloride, or chlorine bleach, may yield false-negative results.

Both EIA and RIA yield definitive, easily interpreted results. In addition, they are more sensitive than TLC techniques, and EIA may be performed in the office or workplace. However, they do not detect as many different drugs as TLC and are more expensive.

The most common EIA tests for identifying marijuana are the EMIT-st (single test) and EMIT d.a.u. (which also identifies several other drugs of abuse), both of which are manufactured by Syva Corporation. EMIT identifies urine concentrations of THC as low as 200 ng/ml with an accuracy of 95%; the EMIT d.a.u. identifies 50 ng/ml concentrations with 95 percent accuracy. The manufacturer recommends a cutoff level of 100 ng/ml for the EMIT d.a.u., to minimize the possibility of reporting a positive result from passive inhalation of marijuana smoke. The 5% of test results that are inaccurate primarily consist of false negatives rather than false positives.[1-3]

Gas Chromatography/Mass Spectrometry

Because of the limitations inherent in TLC and immunoassay methods, they are best used as initial screens. Often greater accuracy will be required—for example, in employee drug-testing programs, where results not only have serious economic implications for the subject but also may have to withstand legal challenge. In such cases, positive results should be confirmed by gas chromatography (GC) or, better yet, by gas chromatography/mass spectrometry (GC/MS).

In GC, the urine sample is heated until it vaporizes. The vapor passes through a column of absorbent material, where individual components are separated and identified by a GC detector according to their chemical and physical properties. GC/MS uses mass spectrometry to analyze the components. GC/MS offers virtually 100 percent accuracy. However, the cost is high—ranging from about $40 per test for volume work to $100 or more for an isolated test.[1]

Measurement of THCA

Blood levels of THC are very low—as low as 1 to 2 ng/ml 24 hours after ingestion—making detection difficult. Although urine levels of THC are even lower (since THC is rapidly biotransformed), one major metabolite is relatively abundant in urine: 11-nor-delta-9-THC-9-carboxylic acid (THCA). Thus, urinalysis is generally the preferred method for detecting marijuana, although blood levels may be more useful in certain situations (see Table 6). For example, blood THC levels are

TABLE 6. Indications for Blood versus Urine Testing for
Marijuana Detection[a]

	Urine	Blood
Diagnosis		
Acute intoxication		x
Marijuana abuse	x	
DUI testing at scene of accident		x
Testing to determine whether admission or mental status evaluation contains drug artifact	x	x
Monitoring of compliance with inpatient substance abuse treatment	x	
Monitoring of compliance with outpatient program	x	
Evaluation of sudden change in mental status or motivation for treatment	x	x
Evaluation of sudden change in mood/behavior/ motivation after return from a pass or visit		x
Screening of visitors to a drug treatment unit	x	
Screening of high risk groups (including adolescents)	x	

[a] Adapted from Verebey K, Gold MS, Mule J: Laboratory testing in the diagnosis of marijuana intoxication and withdrawal. *Psych Ann* 1986;16(4):235–241.

a very good measure for driving-under-the-influence applications.

THCA provides a reliable guide for establishing marijuana use in a patient. For acute users, it can detect use of marijuana as far back as 4 to 6 days before the sample was collected. In chronic users it can detect use that occurred as early as 20 to 30 days prior to sample collection. (The difference is primarily due to the lipid solubility of cannabinoids and the manner in which they are released over time from lipid tissues; see Chapter 2.)

Which Method?

Although TLC of urine samples can detect heavy use of certain drugs, it is not useful for the detection of marijuana use. It is simply not sensitive enough to detect the relatively low levels of THCA present in urine.

Thus, if marijuana use is suspected, the physician must specifically order marijuana screening of the sample. *A "negative" urine sample analyzed by TLC does not rule out recent marijuana use.**

EMIT, RIA, and GC/MS, by contrast, all can reliably detect THCA levels in urine samples. EMIT is a practical method for high-volume automated analysis, because no extraction of THCA or other cannabinoids is necessary. RIA is also useful for screening purposes. GC/MS, although extremely accurate, is too expensive to be used for routine screening. It serves as an excellent method for confirming EMIT or RIA results.

The EMIT test is sensitive to THCA levels as low as 20 ng/ml; however, the manufacturer's recommendations recently raised the "cut-off" to 100 ng/ml—that is, only levels above 100 ng/ml are considered positive.[1] This recommendation does not reflect any change in the

---

* A relatively new TLC method has proved to be very sensitive and accurate, and is a good choice for confirming EMIT or RIA results. However, it is not suitable for mass screening and should not be confused with the inexpensive TLC tests that are commonly used for drug screening.[5]

technical accuracy of the test; it simply provides the test with a greater margin of error. When used for employment or forensic purposes, it gives the subject an additional "benefit of the doubt."

However, when these tests are used *strictly* for medical purposes—that is, for diagnosis or for monitoring of compliance with a therapeutic program—these concerns are largely irrelevant, and the physician should request that the laboratory use the lower thresholds.

A similar distinction arises regarding whether confirmation of test results by another method are warranted. When test results are used solely for diagnostic or therapeutic purposes, and the physician can be certain that they will remain confidential, then the proven accuracy of EMIT suggests that confirmation may be unnecessary—especially if the results are unequivocal.

However, if there is any chance that the test results will be used for broader purposes—for example, in employment decisions or as evidence in civil or criminal proceedings—then it is best to err on the side of caution. Despite the proven high reliability of screening tests, the legal, economic, or social consequences of a positive result are such that positive EMIT or RIA results should in most cases be confirmed by an even more reliable method, such as GC/MS. Such a policy offers sound protection for the subject of the test as well as the physician and those who may act on the results.

In contrast to EMIT, RIA has a lower sensitivity range of 2 ng/ml to 10 ng/ml, depending on the manufacturer.[1] Although it is more sensitive than EMIT, it is more labor-intensive and costly. Specificity of RIA antibodies differs among manufacturers; various antibodies cross-react differently to cannabinoids other than

THCA that may be present in the sample. Therefore, quantitative results obtained from different RIA methods are not directly comparable.

Reliability

The incidence of false-positive urine tests for marijuana screening has been virtually zero in carefully controlled studies.[6,7] Double-blind studies conducted by the National Institute of Drug Abuse found that the EMIT-ST had no false positives and the EMIT-DAU had a false-positive rate of 0.7%.[6]

Verebey conducted a study of 803 urine samples, 40 of which were negative for marijuana.[7] The BPA/TLC method (Verebey 14) correctly identified 97.8% of the samples, with no false positives. In addition, data from the Centers for Disease Control indicate 97 percent reliability for EMIT.[4]

Studies in which EMIT results were confirmed by RIA, BPA/TLC and GC/MS show virtually 100% agreement among all four methods when they are conducted by well-trained technicians following research-quality methods.[4,8] Studies of cross-reactivity with other drugs has not shown them to cause false-positive EMIT results.[9,10] In one study, passive inhalation has resulted in measureable levels of THCA in the urine of a few subjects, but only under extreme conditions, such as confinement in a very small unventilated room with high ambient levels of marijuana smoke.[7] In addition, the urine samples of passive smokers were positive only for a few hours after exposure, and blood samples were uniformly negative. (Strictly speaking, detection of passive inhalation is not a problem of test reliability; in such cases the tests are indeed measuring what they are designed to measure: THC levels. The question of *how* the cannabinoids were introduced into the body—whether ingestion was intentional or incidental—is obviously beyond the scope of laboratory analysis.)

Salivary Analysis

Blood and urine tests for marijuana have their limitations. For example, they fail to provide a good measurement of how recently marijuana use occurred. Analysis of the THC content of saliva by radioimmunoassay can be used to determine when cannabinoids were last smoked.

THC is not secreted into saliva; rather, its presence arises from surface attachment of the substances to oral mucosa. Thus, salivary analysis does *not* directly reflect systemic absorption of marijuana; indeed, THC levels in saliva do not correlate well with THC blood levels or behavioral effects.[1] The role of such tests are, therefore, complementary to other tests, serving only to indicate a time frame of marijuana use. They are most useful when blood tests are unavailable. A positive urine analysis for THCA confirms marijuana use at any time between an hour to four weeks. Positive salivary levels of THC, however, narrows the range down to the twelve-hour period immediately preceding collection of the sample.[1]

Testing Errors

Although marijuana screening tests are highly reliable when performed by well-trained technicians, testing errors can yield incorrect results even when the test itself is technically sound. For example, samples may be adulterated, collected or stored improperly, or mislabeled. Test results may be misread, improperly recorded, or incorrectly reported.

Such errors cannot be entirely eliminated. They can, however, be minimized. Perhaps most important is to use a good laboratory—one that is accredited and, ideally, one with which the physician has had good experience in the past.

It is also important that proper collection and handling methods be followed. Collection should be supervised to prevent adulteration or switching of samples. A first void sample is preferred. To further detect adulteration, the sample should be evaluated immediately after collection for color, temperature, and specific gravity.

THCA breaks down at room temperature in as little as four days; thus, delays in testing may yield false-negative results or underreporting of THCA levels. Samples refrigerated at 4°C or frozen at −20°C have shown no evidence of breakdown after three weeks of storage.[9]

When results will be used for forensic or employment purposes, it is important to maintain the proper "chain of evidence" procedures. Basically, this means that all persons involved in the collection, transport, and testing of the sample are accounted for. Without this accountability, the results will not be admissible in court. Local law enforcement officials or legal counsel may be consulted for the proper forms and methods used to verify the chain of custody.

In light of the potential for testing errors, positive drug results should be confirmed, if at all possible, by testing of a second sample. In cases where it may be difficult to obtain a timely second sample—for example, in a case where driving-under-the-influence is suspected—the initial sample should be divided into two *before* it is sent to the laboratory. If marijuana use is strongly suspected, both samples can be sent out immediately for independent analysis. For screening programs, the second sample can simply be stored until the first test results are returned. At that time, the second sample can be used to confirm a positive result; if, on the other hand, the initial test result is negative, the second sample can be discarded.

References

1. Gold MS, Bensinger PB (eds): *The Complete Guide to Drug Testing.* New York, Random House, 1987.
2. Schwartz RH, Hayden GF. Riddile M: Laboratory detection of marijuana use. *Am J Child Dis* 1985;139:1093–1096.
3. Schwartz RH, Hawks RL: Laboratory detection of marijuana use. *JAMA* 1985;254:788–792.
4. Verebey K, Gold MS, Mule J: Laboratory testing in the diagnosis of marijuana intoxication and withdrawal. *Psych Ann* 1986;16(4):235–241.
5. Kogan MJ, Newman E, Willson NJ: Detection of marijuana metabolite 11-nor-delta-9-carboxylic acid in human urine by bonded phase absorption thin-layer chromatography. *J Chromatogr* 1984;306:441–443.
6. Gorodetzky CW, Cone EJ, Johnson RE: Validity of EMIT and

RIA for detection in urine of marijuana cigarette smoking. *Pharmacologist* 1983;25–27.

7. Verebey K, Jukofsky D, Mule SJ: Evaluation of a new TLC confirmation technique for positive EMIT cannabinoid urine samples. *Res Comm Substance Abuse* 1985;6:1–9.

8. Kogan MJ, Alrazi J, Pearson DJ, et al: The confirmation of SYVA EMIT dau and Roche Abusescreen RIA (I-125) urine cannabinoid immunoassays by GC/MS and bonded phase absorption-TLC methods of assay. *J Forensic Sci* 1986;31:494–500.

9. Sutheimer CA, Yarborough K, Helper BR, et al: Detection and confirmation of urinary cannabinoids. *J Anal Toxicol* 1985;9:156–160.

10. El Sohly MA, Jones AB, El Sohly HN, et al: Analysis of the major metabolite of delta-9-tetrahydrocannabinol in urine. VI. Specificity of the assay with respect to indole carboxylic acids. *J Anal Toxicol* 1985;9:190–191.

7

Treatment of Marijuana Abuse

Treatment of addiction, including marijuana addiction, is a highly specialized field, and a consultation from qualified specialists should be sought when a diagnosis or tentative diagnosis of marijuana addiction is established. In many cases the patient will undergo detoxification within a substance abuse program, with the family physician coordinating ongoing treatment and monitoring in close conjunction with the specialist. After detoxification, the patient will require extensive counseling and, in most cases, medical supervision.

The particulars of this treatment will, of course, vary according to the treatment program and the patient's own needs, but the program should embrace a number of fundamental considerations. A keystone of our approach to treatment is recognition of the biochemical basis of addiction in general and marijuana addiction in particular. Successful treatment is built on the concept that the patient is suffering from a *physiological* disorder, not from a personality disorder or moral failing.

A number of factors reinforce the idea that the marijuana addict suffers from a biochemical disorder that amplifies the drug's reinforcing properties. Among non-addicted marijuana users, the drug is usually used in *response* to a failure to cope with some type of stress—for example, interpersonal, economic, or scholastic. Among marijuana addicts, however, we have found that *marijuana reinforces its own use.*[1] Although the addict may begin using marijuana initially in response to psychosocial stressors, the presence of these stressors is not necessary to maintain the addiction. Marijuana addicts will continue to use the drug even if the initial psychosocial stressors are removed or mitigated.

Disease Concept

As with all addictions, it is essential to approach marijuana addiction from a *medical* perspective rather than a *moral* one. Family members, employers—sometimes even the patient—will usually define the addiction as a moral failing. They may see marijuana addiction as a mysterious and metaphysical affliction rather than a medical problem, and believe that the addict is irresponsible and unmotivated. A common misperception is that the addict has brought his or her problems on him- or herself and can overcome them if only by exercising enough willpower.

Unfortunately, the term *willpower* does more to obscure the issues than to clarify them, for it falsely assumes that all individuals have a similar capacity to resist temptations. For a susceptible individual to resist a marijuana addiction would require as much "willpower" as a chef on a hunger strike.

Current medical evidence supports the idea that marijuana addiction is a primary disease of the mind and nervous system.[2-10] The problem is not insufficient willpower, but rather initially trying the drug plus an abnormal sensitivity to marijuana's reinforcing properties.

When explaining these facts to the patient and family, it is important that they not be left with the impression that the addict's desire and effort to overcome the addiction are unimportant. In other words, the physician must emphasize that biology is not destiny. He or she must be careful that explanations of the addiction's biochemical basis do not become the basis of a rationalization for not doing anything about it.

The message, rather, is that while ''   nt's own desire—"will"—to get better is essen.   uccessful treatment, *willpower alone is not enough*.   r words, the patient must overcome the addiction,   e or she cannot do it on his or her own.

Fundamentals of Treatment

The basic model for treatment of marijuan. tion, like alcoholism, is initial detoxification follov. lifelong abstinence. Unfortunately, the physician. few pharmacologic options to help these patients, ё the case with clonidine for narcotic detoxification a. naltrexone for prevention of narcotics relapse.

Treatment is a long and often frustrating process for the physician as well as the patient, and therapeutic failures are common. Treatment may be complicated by the presence of concurrent substance-abuse problems, which is common among such patients.[1] The patient will typically exhibit denial, deception, and hostility toward the physician; these behaviors, coupled with the attitudes of the family, often make it difficult for the physician to remain objective.

Treatment programs vary. Whatever the program that is selected, we recommend that it include the following model program characteristics:

- It should have a philosophical basis that includes no use of marijuana, alcohol, or other drugs. Programs that offer psychotherapy or other interventions while the individual continues to abuse drugs simply prolong the addictive process by giving the patient and family the illusion of progress.
- It must provide accurate and current information on the current hazards of drug abuse.
- It must be active in helping the patient overcome his or her addiction and in encouraging changes, rather than relying on lectures or harangues.
- It should be appropriate to the patient's age and background; for example, programs for adolescents should address their interests and special problems.
- It should treat the family as well as the patient. Where the patient is an adolescent, it should include *active* parental involvement. Parents should not feel that their support and setting of

limits is no longer necessary because their child is in a program.

- It should emphasize the present, including the immediate, as well as long-term, damage that the patient suffers from drug abuse.
- It should stress accountability on the part of the patient for his or her actions, and it should not shield the patient from the consequences of destructive behavior.
- It *must* employ reliable urine collection and testing as an objective indicator of compliance and therapeutic success.

The involvement of the family—especially with younger patients—cannot be overemphasized. Our program and many others routinely require an intensive one-week family intervention. There is a high incidence of coexisting patterns of drug and/or alcohol abuse among parents and siblings of adolescent addicts. This factor contributes to the problem of denial, and typically promotes continued use. In some cases, parents have actually subsidized the adolescent's drug habit, knowingly or not. In addition, families may often permit themselves to be held as "emotional hostages," out of a mistaken belief that confrontation will lead to greater drug use or other self-destructive behaviors. These types of dysfunctional behaviors are commonly seen among families of substance abusers, and they must be addressed. To return the patient—especially an adolescent patient—to such a home without a change in these patterns is simply setting the stage for continued drug use.

History and Physical

The first step is a thorough history and physical examination, including a neurological examination if it is indicated by the presentation. In addition, extensive laboratory testing is necessary to identify any medical, neurologic, or psychiatric deficits, as well as to identify any other possible causes behind the patient's symptoms. Tests should include complete blood count (CBC), liver and renal functions, and electrolytes. Serologic analysis and urinalysis should be performed to detect the presence of additional drugs. Evaluation of neuroendocrine function, including dexamethasone suppression and thyroid stimulation tests, may be indicated for coexisting psychiatric, neurological, and medical problems.[4]

Detoxification

The next step in the treatment of marijuana addiction is acute detoxification. Fortunately, this step is among the easiest. Withdrawal symptoms are mild, provided the patient is not suffering from concurrent dependencies on other drugs such as alcohol or cocaine.

A variety of treatment approaches have been devised.[1] Severe cases may require an initial phase of hospitalization and specific inpatient treatment. Hospitalization is a powerful intervention; it interrupts the "cycle of addiction" and permits the addict to confront denials and rationalizations. Moreover, it disrupts the social and environmental cues that serve to reinforce the use of marijuana. In addition, it establishes a controlled environment in which careful medical, neurological, and psychiatric evaluation can take place, and it helps ensure abstinence through the critical first phase of treatment.[1] Outpatient treatment is appropriate for less severe forms of cannabis dependence where the course of addiction has been neither long nor serious and the patient's support system is strong. Additional drug problems, however, tend to undermine outpatient treatment.[1]

Treatment Program Elements

Both inpatient and outpatient programs may include a number of the following elements[11]:

- Group therapy, the most common type, may be task oriented or confrontational. They help the patient gain perspective on the problem by exposing him or her to others with similar problems under the guidance of a trained counselor. In addition, the group can help the patient gain socialization, communication, and problem-solving skills.
- Family therapy, as noted above, is essential to ultimate success of the treatment. Its focus is on communication among family members as well as development of self-awareness and insight into dysfunctional behaviors.
- Individual therapy may be an option for patients who require specialized care or who are reluctant to participate in group therapy.
- Education is an important part of therapy, helping to dispel the myths and rationalizations that perpetuate addiction.

Behavioral therapy uses techniques such as aversive conditioning and contingency contracting to treat addiction. As with most behavioral techniques, consistent results are difficult to achieve once the patient leaves the controlled (that is, inpatient) setting; the fundamental drawback is that in the real world, drugs are by far the most powerful reinforcer in the patient's life. Even so, these techniques may be a useful adjunct to other forms of therapy. Aversive conditioning, in which unpleasant associations are linked with drug use (e.g., induction of vomiting after ingestion of drugs), has little long-term utility, presumably because the aversive stimuli are not present outside of the controlled treatment environment. Contingency contracting involves a formal contract between the patient and therapist, in which specific consequences for continued drug use are agreed to. Unfortunately, patients may refuse to honor or renew these contracts once they leave the inpatient facility.

Counseling and Follow-Up

Marijuana dependence, like alcoholism, is a chronic addiction associated with progressive deterioration. As with alcoholism, there is no cure; the only treatment is lifelong abstinence. An extensive counseling program, under the supervision of a qualified substance abuse specialist, is indicated.

For both the patient and family, a 12-step program modeled on Alcoholics Anonymous (for the patient) and Al-Anon (for families) is extremely useful (Figure 2).

The Twelve Steps

1. We admitted we were powerless over alcohol—that our lives had become unmanageable.

2. Came to believe that a Power greater than ourselves could restore us to sanity.

3. Made a decision to turn our will and our lives over to the care of God *as we understood him.*

4. Made a searching and fearless personal inventory of ourselves.

5. Admitted to God, to ourselves and to another human being the exact nature of our wrongs.

6. Were entirely ready to have God remove all these defects of character.

7. Humbly asked him to remove our shortcomings.

8. Made a list of all persons we had harmed, and became willing to make amends to them all.

9. Made direct amends to such people wherever possible, except when to do so would injure them or others.

10. Continued to take personal inventory and when we were wrong promptly admitted it.

11. Sought through prayer and meditation to improve our conscious contact with God *as we understood Him,* praying only for knowledge of His will for us and the power to carry that out.

12. Having had a spiritual awakening as the result of these Steps, we tried to carry this message to others, and to practice these principles in all our affairs.

FIGURE 2. The Twelve Steps, originally developed by Alcoholics Anonymous, have been adapted by many other self-help groups, including those for people suffering from a variety of drug dependencies. Reprinted with permission of Alcoholics Anonymous World Services, Incorporated.

Peer groups modeled on these programs include Narcotics Anonymous and Naranon; others may exist locally and can be identified with the help of substance-abuse specialists or social-service agencies. Participation in these groups should be an adjunct to treatment, not a substitute for it. Significantly greater treatment success rates have been achieved by instituting inpatient or outpatient treatment concurrently with such programs.[4,6,12] Evidence of success should be monitored by gathering feedback from patients, their family, their friends, their employers, *and always* their urine.

Prognosis

The likelihood of success depends to a great extent on the individual. Patients with mild addiction and strong motivation to be drug free usually do well. Equally important are sociological factors. A person who functioned well before their involvement with marijuana will usually function well after treatment. A history of steady employment or good grades and strong support from the family are good predictors of successful treatment.

More problematic are patients with poor support systems and a history of social/psychological dysfunction. In these cases treatment of the addiction alone is likely to be futile; a broad program of treatment and counseling must be developed. For these patients therapy is long and difficult, and the chances of success are less.

References

1. Miller NS, Gold MS: Marijuana (cannabis) dependence (addiction) and consequences. *J Substance Abuse* (in press, 1988).
2. American Medical Association: AMA labels marijuana a dangerous drug. *Psychiatric News* 1981(Apr 17):1.
3. American Medical Association Council on Scientific Affairs: Marijuana. *JAMA* 1981;246:1823–1827.
4. Dackis CA, Gold MS, Estroff TW: Inpatient treatment of addiction, in *APA Manual of Therapeutics*. Washington, DC, American Psychiatric Assocation (in press).
5. Harris LS, Dewey WL, Razdan RK: Cannabis: Its chemistry, pharmacology, and toxicology, in, Martin WR (ed), *Drug Addiction*. Berlin, Springer-Verlag, 1977.
6. Jones RT, Benzowitz N, Bachman JA: Clinical studies of cannabis tolerance and dependence. *Ann NY Acad Sci* 1976;282:221–239.
7. Negrete JC: Symptoms of cannabis intoxication in a group of users. *Toxicomanics* 1974;7:7–18.
8. Negrete JC: Psychiatric effects of cannabis use, in Fehr KO, Kalant H (eds), *Adverse Health and Behavioral Consequences of Cannabis Use*. Working papers for the ARF/WHO Scientific Meeting, Toronto, 1981.
9. Tinklenberg JR (ed) *Marijuana and Health Hazards*. New York, Academic, 1975.
10. Estroff TW, Gold MS: Psychiatric presentations of marijuana abuse. *Psychiatric Annals* 1986;16(4):221–224.
11. Schnoll SH, Daghestani AN: Treatment of marijuana abuse. *Psych Ann* 1986;16(4):249–254.
12. Johnston ID, O'Malley PM, Bachman JA: Use of licit and illicit drugs by America's high school students: National trends, 1975–1984. [DHHS publication no. (ADM) 85-1394.] Washington, DC, U.S. Government Printing Office, 1985.

8

Prevention of Marijuana Abuse

Treatment of marijuana addiction is difficult, and success rates tend to be low. A preferable approach is to prevent drug abuse at the outset.

But do efforts at prevention work? The evidence of recent years suggests that they do. Drug use among adolescents has fallen dramatically in recent years (with the exception of cocaine). Although many factors undoubtedly contribute to this trend—such as the increased conservatism of the youthful population—it is probably no accident that prevention programs have proliferated during the same time period. (Incidentally, similar trends are evident in the campaigns against smoking and drunk driving.) The key to the success of these recent programs appears to be *accurate information* that avoids both the hysteria of early prevention efforts (which portrayed risks in ways that were obviously untrue) and the drug-culture myth of marijuana as a perfectly safe drug.

For the family physician, prevention efforts should take a two-pronged approach. On one hand, it involves identification of at-risk individuals, face-to-face education with them and their families, and appropriate interventions. Just as important, however, are community education efforts. Although some physicians may be uncomfortable taking a high-profile role in community drug-prevention efforts, physicians' participation is especially appropriate. Traditionally, leadership in public-health issues has fallen to physicians by virtue of their authority, background, and standing within the community. Just as physicians in an earlier era worked to eliminate the conditions responsible for outbreaks of infectious disease or unsafe working conditions, so should today's physician help guide efforts to prevent drug abuse, one of the leading public-health problems of our time.

Historical Perspectives

Early attempts at prevention were based on the idea that adolescents tried drugs because they were ignorant of their consequences. Often these prevention efforts contained messages intended to create fear of drugs. However, these messages were often so extreme that they lacked credibility, especially among those who had some familiarity with the drugs and their effects.[1]

Later research revealed the importance of interpersonal and intrapersonal factors—attitudes, beliefs, and values—in the decision to experiment with drugs.[2]

These findings led to an "affective" approach, which attempted to prevent drug abuse by addressing these underlying factors. Other programs stressed alternative activities, such as sports, to replace peer-related drug-abuse behavior and to reduce alienation.

Although these affective approaches may be beneficial in a general way, they have not proved effective in preventing drug abuse.[3,4] Current efforts, by contrast, are aimed not only at providing education, but also at developing the psychosocial skills necessary to resist peer pressure and other social and environmental influences. This is the underlying rationale for the "Just Say No" efforts. However, to be effective, we must do more than simply teach children to say no; we must teach them *how* to say no. We must give them accurate information, but we must also give them the tools that will enable them to make use of this information. Role-playing and discussion groups are just two of the techniques that can help children learn to make their own informed and rational decisions.

In their summary of relevant research, Battjes and Jones identify the following general implications for prevention[5]:

- Because of the diversity of drug abuse problems, no single solution represents a panacea. Prevention programs must be targeted to specific populations and specific drug-use behaviors.
- Because drug use is strongly influenced by social and environmental factors, programs aimed at developing the skills to resist such influences (for example, the "Just Say No" campaign) are appropriate. For certain groups however—such as

early and late initiators—other psychiatric or behavioral disorders may play a larger role and must be addressed.

- Programs aimed at adolescents must take into account the "normal developmental challenges" of adolescence. For example, given the prevalence of risk-taking behavior among adolescents, a program that redirects this behavior is likely to be more successful than one that ignores it or attempts to eliminate it altogether.
- Preventive programs should begin early, well before age 15.
- Some research suggests that prevention of alcohol and tobacco use may help prevent marijuana use, although this assumption has not been tested rigorously.
- Drug information may be an appropriate tactic, but it should be combined with teaching of the social skills necessary to resist peer pressure. Information should be presented by "credible senders," should be relevant to the target, should address the audience's values, and should be appropriate to the audience's developmental level.

Family-Oriented Prevention Efforts

Risk Factors for Marijuana Abuse

For individual families and patients, prevention efforts begin with identification of those who are at risk of substance abuse. (See Table 7.) The indicators out-

TABLE 7. Factors Influencing the Likelihood of Drug Abuse

Predisposing factors
   Parental alcohol or drug problems
   Divorce, money problems, or other sources of family stress
   Perceived use of drugs by siblings or friends
   Poor parent–child communication
   Access to marijuana
   Preexisting psychological or behavioral problems
   Extensive peer involvement
Preventive factors
   Accurate and authoritative information about drugs and their risks
   Early intervention

lined in Chapter 5 are some of the most common factors that we have seen accompanying marijuana abuse. Obviously these factors do not *cause* drug abuse, but they can alert the physician to underlying problems that may predispose the patient to experiment with drugs. For example, an adolescent whose grades drop suddenly but who tests negative for marijuana or other drugs may be suffering from undiagnosed depression, and may eventually turn to drugs as a conscious or unconscious attempt at self-medication.

A key risk factor for drug abuse is the family's attitudes toward drugs—not only illicit drugs such as marijuana and cocaine, but also such substances as alcohol, cigarettes, and even caffeine. One of the most significant warning signs is a parent who suffers from chemical dependency or other compulsive/addictive disorders. Indeed, family values as a whole play an important part in determining an adolescent's perspective on drugs. This is not to say that parental use of alcohol or other substances will necessarily lead to drug problems by children. More important is *how* these substances are used—or abused. More broadly, it is important to look at how families deal with problems and stress in general. If, for example, a parent uses alcohol as an escape mechanism, he or she sends a clear signal to the child about the appropriateness of such behavior. Similarly, if a parent drinks coffee compulsively, the child tends to accept as normal all forms of compulsive behavior.

Another factor is a poor relationship between the parents and child. It is often difficult for the physician to uncover dysfunctional family dynamics, at least until some other problem brings it to his or her attention. A careful history-taking of *all* family members will often offer some clues, but they may be subtle. Other signs may be apparent in parent–child interactions during an office visit, or from the parent's interactions with the physician. Major family stresses—divorce, a death in the family, money problems—can trigger drug use not only for adolescents but for parents as well.

A longitudinal study of psychotropic drug use among adolescents and young adults yields important insights about who is at risk for marijuana dependency.[6] In the study, the rate of marijuana use rose from the preteen ages to about age 18. From age 18 to ages 23 or 24, the rate of use stabilizes, and drops dramatically thereafter. The pattern was virtually identical for females and males, although the rate of use was consistently lower among girls (Figure 3).

The study also revealed that current use of alcohol and cigarettes are significant risk factors for initiation among marijuana use. Among the males in the study, prior use of alcohol was also a significant risk factor.

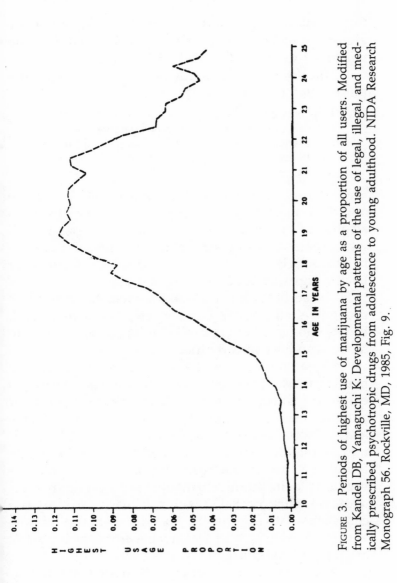

FIGURE 3. Periods of highest use of marijuana by age as a proportion of all users. Modified from Kandel DB, Yamaguchi K: Developmental patterns of the use of legal, illegal, and medically prescribed psychotropic drugs from adolescence to young adulthood. NIDA Research Monograph 56. Rockville, MD, 1985, Fig. 9.

Other risk factors include age (those younger than 20 are at the highest risk of initiating marijuana use) and perceived use of marijuana by friends.

The authors of this study note some important implications for preventing drug abuse:

> Early prevention efforts targeted toward reducing young people's initiation into the use of cigarettes and/or alcohol would reduce the use of marijuana, and prevention of early marijuana use would reduce involvement in other illicit drugs.[6]

They note further that the link between marijuana use and other illicit drugs is stronger than the link between alcohol or cigarettes and marijuana. In other words, while some adolescents use marijuana even if they have never used cigarettes or alcohol, virtually none use other illicit drugs without first using marijuana.

The authors also note that their results suggest that preventive efforts will be more effective if they reach those who have not yet used marijuana, as opposed to those who have already tried it.

Kaplan found a number of predictors of increased marijuana use: Those who initially use marijuana at an early age, during a time of psychological distress, or without peer motivation are more likely to become heavy users.[7] Adverse consequences of initial use diminish the likelihood of escalated use. Another study found that use of marijuana by peers is a significant predictor for initiation into marijuana use.[8] Peer involvement is highly correlated with marijuana use.[9] Adolescents who date extensively, spend a great deal of time with their friends, and feel remote from their parents are more likely to use marijuana.[10]

Another factor is the degree of parental monitoring.

Those with low-parental monitoring are at increased risk of developing drug problems.[11] The same study showed that the child's peer group was also a significant predictor of marijuana use.

Teaching Parents to Identify Marijuana Use

It is important to routinely assess parents' knowledge of drug problems and their awareness of their children's activities. There is currently an epidemic of substance abuse in the United States, and most children will be exposed to it sooner or later. It is therefore vital for parents as well as practitioners to be aware of signals of actual or potential drug abuse. If necessary, parents should also be given some clear instructions on what to do—and what not to do—if they suspect that their child *is* using marijuana or other drugs. Stress to them that although drug abuse is a big problem, it is not one they have to face alone. Physicians, counselors, and volunteer groups can all help provide the guidance and support that is needed.

Above all, it is important to stress *early intervention*. Ideally, intervention should be aimed at preventing the problem altogether rather than treat it. But even when treatment is necessary, it is more successful early in the course of addiction, before new behavioral and social patterns become deeply ingrained. It is, therefore, doubly important that parents be able to recognize signs of *potential* drug abuse as well as actual abuse. A good rule of thumb for parents is: When in doubt, call the family doctor.

Parents should also receive some guidance about how to approach their children concerning drug abuse.

Naturally, parents want to avoid false accusations or an undermining of their children's trust, but they must understand that inaction can be deadly. Suggest that they call you rather than confront the child directly if they suspect that their child is abusing drugs, or if they are concerned that their child is headed toward a drug problem. This approach is an emotionally safer course than direct confrontation, and it permits the parent and physician to develop a rational approach to the problem.

In many cases it makes sense for someone other than the parent—such as the physician or guidance counselor—to initially confront the adolescent who may be using marijuana or other drugs. Doing so can help direct any feelings of anger, betrayal, and rebellion away from the parent, and may permit a more rational discussion of the risks and consequences of drug use. This strategy is especially useful where the history reveals dysfunctional family relationships.

This is not to say, however, that parents can abdicate their responsibilities. Once the confrontational phase is over, the parents must establish and enforce appropriate limits and expectations for the child. It is important to emphasize to parents that successful prevention or treatment will largely depend on the home environment.

Community Prevention Efforts

Resources

In the past several years, the problem of drug abuse has gained widespread attention, and a number of organizations have formed to address the problems of drugs in the community. These groups can serve as both a resource and a model for community drug-prevention programs. Table 8 lists some of the better-known organizations, and information on how to get in touch with them.

A Model Program for Schools and Communities

As noted above, the physician's role in community prevention efforts is vital. Often the physician can serve as a catalyst for action, and provide the expertise and information needed for an effective program. The time demands need not be great; far more important is the "moral support" and encouragement that the physician can lend to concerned parents, teachers, and civic leaders.

A strong community effort can include the following elements:

- Peer efforts
- Speakers
- Information bureau
- Discussion groups
- Alternatives
- School programs

School Programs

In 1986, the U.S. Department of Education published a model program for eliminating drugs from schools.[12] It outlines a 12-point approach (Table 9), with specific suggestions and case histories of schools where

TABLE 8. Drug Prevention Organizations and Resources[a]

American Council for Drug Education, Inc. 5820 Hubbard Drive, Rockville, MD 20852. A membership organization; offers "Marijuana: A Second Look," a kit for physicians and schools; as well as "Building Drug-Free Schools," a four-part drug-prevention kit for schools K–12. Includes three written guides and a film. ACDE also offers films and other materials.

Boy Scouts of America. 1325 Walnut Hill Lane, Irving, TX 75038-3096. Offers information on drug abuse prevention as part of law-enforcement Explorers.

Californians for Drug-Free Youth. P.O. Box 1758, Thousand Oaks, CA 91360. An umbrella organization for more than 350 parent groups in California.

Department of Education, Office of the Secretary. Room 4181, 400 Maryland Avenue S.W., Washington, D.C. 20202. Provides grant funds, distributes information, and helps coordinate local prevention efforts.

Families in Action. Suite 300 3845 North Druid Hills Road, Decatur, GA 30033. The first of many nationwide Families in Action groups, this group serves as an example and mentor for programs nationwide, and distributes a guide for forming similar groups.

"Just Say No" Clubs. Pacific Institute for Research and Evaluation. 177 N. California Blvd., Suite 200, Walnut Creek, CA 94596. Provides information on "Just Say No" clubs worldwide, as well as on how to start a club.

National Clearinghouse for Drug Abuse Information. ADAMHA, Office of Substance Abuse and Prevention, 5600 Fishers Lane, Rockville, MD 20857. Provides free pamphlets and other information.

National Institute on Drug Abuse. ADAMHA, 5600 Fishers Lane, Rockville, MD 20857. The Institute sponsors and conducts research on drug abuse and prevention.

National Federation of Parents for Drug-Free Youth (NFP). 8730 Georgia Ave., Suite 200, Silver Spring, MD 20910. An 8,000-member organization, NFP publishes newsletters and makes other information available.

Ohio Federation of Families for Drug-Free Youth. 80 South 6th Street, Columbus, OH 43215. Affiliated with NFP; works with parents and youths to promote drug-free life-styles.

TABLE 8. (cont.)

PRIDE (Parent Resources Institute on Drug Education. Robert W. Woodruff Volunteer Services). 100 Edgewood Avenue, Suite 1216, Atlanta, GA 30303. (404) 658-2548/1-800-241-9746. Offers books, pamphlets, films, and other resources for drug education.

Responsible Adolescents Can Help (REACH). 8730 Georgia Ave., Suite 200, Silver Spring, MD 20910. An outgrowth of NFP, REACH provides information on how to set up training seminars, as well as other related information.

Students to Offset Peer Pressure (STOPP). Consulting Services. P.O. Box 103, Hudson, NH 03051. Provides information on starting local STOPP clubs.

Texans' War on Drugs. 7800 Shoal Creek Blvd., Suite 381-W, Austin, TX 78757. A statewide drug abuse prevention organization that has become a national model. Provides guidelines and assistance to other states and nations.

Tough Love. Community Service Foundation, Box 70, Sellersville, PA 18960. A network of parent groups for families with children involved with drugs.

Virginia Beach Council of PTAs. Juvenile Protection Committee, 213 Brentwood Crescent, Virginia Beach, VA 23452. Developed Courtwatch, a computerized docket of drug-related court cases.

World Youth Against Drugs. 100 Edgewood Avenue, Suite 1002, Atlanta, GA 30303. Publishes a quarterly newsletter that reaches an audience in more than 35 countries. Also has a pen-pal network for sharing ideas on fighting drug abuse.

Youth to Youth/CompDrug. 700 Bryden Road, Columbus, OH 43215. A prevention (as opposed to treatment) program; offers seminars.

Youth Who Care. P.O. Box 4074, Grand Junction, CO 81502. An offshoot of the state's Parents Who Care organization.

---

[a] Prevention, Cooperation, Enforcement: Mobilizing Against Illegal Drugs. Washington, DC: United States Information Agency, 1987.

TABLE 9. A Plan for Achieving Schools without Drugs

Parents
1. Teach standards of right and wrong, and demonstrate these standards through personal example.
2. Help children to resist peer pressure to use drugs by supervising their activities, knowing who their friends are, and talking with them about their interests and problems.
3. Be knowledgeable about drugs and signs of drug use. When symptoms are observed, respond promptly.

Schools
4. Determine the extent and character of drug use and establish a means of monitoring that use regularly.
5. Establish clear and specific rules regarding drug use that include strong corrective actions.
6. Enforce established policies against drug use fairly and consistently. Implement security measures to eliminate drugs on school premises and at school functions.
7. Implement a comprehensive drug prevention curriculum for kindergarten through grade 12, teaching that drug use is wrong and harmful and supporting and strengthening resistance to drugs.
8. Reach out to the community for support and assistance in making the school's antidrug policy and program work. Develop collaborative arrangements in which school personnel, parents, school boards, law enforcement officers, treatment organizations, and private groups can work together to provide necessary resources.

Students
9. Learn about the effects of drug use, the reasons why drugs are harmful, and ways to resist pressures to try drugs.
10. Use an understanding of the danger posed by drugs to help other students avoid them. Encourage other students to resist drugs, persuade those using drugs to seek help, and report those selling drugs to parents and the school principal.

TABLE 9. *(cont.)*

Communities
11. Help schools fight drugs by providing them with the expertise and financial resources of community groups and agencies.
12. Involve local law enforcement agencies in all aspects of drug prevention: assessment, enforcement, and education. The police and courts should have well-established and mutually supportive relationships with the schools.

SOURCE: U.S. Department of Education. *What Works: Schools Without Drugs.* U.S. Department of Education, 1986.

drug use has been curtailed successfully. Another school program has been developed by the American Council for Drug Education (5820 Hubbard Drive, Rockville, MD 20852; telephone (301) 984-5700). Consisting of a film and three written guides, the program discusses school policies, a model curriculum, and community efforts.

One of the most important of its recommendations—and one that physicians can play an important part in—is education, beginning at the earliest possible ages. Children may be exposed to illicit drugs, including marijuana, during the first few years of school (or even before, if the parents use drugs in their presence). Because education must precede exposure for maximum effect, it should begin as early as possible.

Physicians can help develop antidrug curricula, and may speak to classes or school assemblies. The message may also be incorporated into talks about medicine in general—for example, at a "career day" for high school students. Although the information must, of course, be tailored to the appropriate educational and developmental level, it should be factual, supported by examples and research, and specific. Even young students may show surprising sophistication, and it is important not to appear to be "talking down" to them. An initial question-and-answer session can help gauge students' knowledge and experience.

References

1. Bell CS, Battjes RJ: Overview of drug abuse prevention research. NIDA Research Monograph Series 63. Prevention research: Deterring drug abuse among children and adolescents, 1985.
2. Goodstadt MS: Impact and roles of drug information in drug education. *J Drug Educ* 1975;5:223–233.
3. Blum RH, Garfield EF, Johnstone JL, Magistad JG: Drug education: Further results and recommendations. *J Drug Issues* 1978;8:379–426.
4. Schaps E, Di Bartolo R, Moskowitz J, Palley CS, Churgin S: A review of 127 drug abuse prevention program evaluations. *J Drug Issues* 1981;11:17–43.
5. Battjes RJ, Jones CL: *Implications of etiological research for preventive interventions and future research.* NIDA Research Monograph Series 56. Rockville, MD, 1985:269–276.
6. Kandel DB, Yamaguchi K: *Developmental patterns of the use of legal, illegal, and medically prescribed psychotropic drugs from adolescence to young adulthood.* NIDA Research Monograph Series 56. Rockville, MD, 1985.
7. Kaplan HB, Martin SS, Johnson RJ, Robbins, CA: Escalation of marijuana use: Application of a general theory of deviant behavior. *J Health Soc Behav* 1986;27(Mar)44–61.
8. Yamaguchi K, Kandel DB. Patterns of drug use from adolescence to young adulthood: III. Predictors of progression. *Am J Public Health* 1984;74:673–681.
9. Petersen RC: Marijuana overview, in Glantz MD (ed), *Correlates and Consequences of Marijuana Use.* Rockville, MD, National Institute on Drug Abuse, 1984, p. 4.

10. Johnston LD, Bachman JG, O'Malley PM: Highlights from Student Drug Use in America, 1975–1980. Washington, DC, National Institute on Drug Abuse, 1980 [DHHS publication no. (ADM)82-1208].
11. Dishion TJ, Loeber R: Adolescent marijuana and alcohol use: The role of parents and peers revisited. *Am J Drug Alcohol Abuse* 1985;11(1,2):11–25.
12. U.S. Department of Education: *What Works: Schools Without Drugs*. Washington, DC, U.S. Department of Education, 1986.

APPENDIX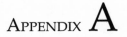

Questions Patients and Parents Ask about Marijuana

Here are some of the questions that physicians may be asked by patients and parents concerning marijuana use, as well as answers presented in layman's terms.

1. What is marijuana?

Marijuana is the dried leaves and flowers of the *cannabis sativa* plant, which grows wild throughout the world and is cultivated in many countries. The most powerful strains of *cannabis sativa* are now grown illegally in the United States.

Adapted from Gold MS: *The Facts About Drugs and Alcohol.* New York, Bantam, 1987. Copyright 1986 by Mark S. Gold, M.D. Used by permission.

2. What is hashish?

Hashish is another, more powerful by-product of the cannabis plant. It is also smoked. Derived from the resinous secretions of the plant, "hash" is mainly produced in the Middle East. Its oils are collected, dried, and then pressed into balls or flat slabs for transport.

3. How are they used?

Marijuana is almost always smoked. The dried leaves are crumpled, cleansed of seeds, and rolled into the shape of a cigarette—the classic "reefer" or "joint." Pot can also be smoked in a water pipe (known as a bong) for a stronger effect. Hashish, like marijuana, is usually smoked—typically in a special pipe.

4. Are there other ways to use these drugs?

Yes. Marijuana and hashish have also been included in a wide variety of baked goods—hash brownies, magic cookies, etc. The effect, while not as strong as smoking, can be potent. Because marijuana will not dissolve in water, it is very rarely injected.

5. How potent are the various forms?

The effects of the different strains of marijuana are directly related to the amount of THC present. On a scale of 1 to 10, marijuana imported from South America in the 1960s had a potency of 1–2, whereas forms of sensimilla grown here or in Asia (e.g., Thai sticks) are ranked above 7.

6. What are the mental effects of smoking marijuana?

No one describes the effects of marijuana exactly the same. In fact, the historical descriptions of marijuana have filled literature for centuries. The "high" that is often described is an intoxicated feeling with a heightened sense of awareness to music, light, and the environment—better known as the "Wow!" effect.

However, the reactions to marijuana vary widely. One reason is variable potency. Another factor is how long someone's been a marijuana user. In addition, the subjective nature of the user's feelings are strongly influenced by the environment. Many users, for example, report paranoia, anxiety, and withdrawal from social interaction as a primary effect.

7. Do people develop a tolerance to marijuana?

The more marijuana you use, the more you need each time to recreate the high. This is because marijuana's active ingredients accumulate rapidly in the body, building tolerance. This causes a decrease in the effect with each repeated dose. Because the amount of THC in marijuana is uncontrolled—unlike alcohol or pills—each dose is different. Thus it's very hard to gauge exactly how much use will cause tolerance and dependence. Some studies have demonstrated that tolerance can develop even after low doses.

8. How does marijuana affect the body?

THC is absorbed through the lungs into the bloodstream almost immediately after smoking. It clings to the fatty linings of the cells. It is then released back into the bloodstream over a period of time, usually a week or so.

Some drugs, such as alcohol and cocaine, are soluble in water. They are expelled from the body relatively quickly. But THC residue remains attached to the fat cells, and it builds up unless no more marijuana is ingested for at least a week. Anyone who smokes marijuana more often than once a week may never rid their body of the drug's effects.

9. Is marijuana harmful?

Yes! The harmful effects of marijuana can occur after any amount of use, but they are more frequent with prolonged use. These problems can include: impairment of eye–hand coordination, which makes driving unsafe; infertility; increased heart rate, which can lead to panic attacks; and distorted visual and time perceptions, leading to anxiety and paranoia. Overdose of marijuana can result in a trance-like state.

Three body systems—the endocrine (glandular) system, the respiratory (breathing) system, and the immune system seem to bear the brunt of marijuana's effect with chronic use. Sore throats and upper respiratory ailments such as bronchitis are common. The tar in marijuana is five to ten times greater than that in cigarettes, thus increasing the already dangerous risk of cancer for pot-smoking smokers.

Recent studies show that marijuana also reduces the efficiency of the body's immune system. Marijuana smokers have more infections and are less protected against illness from bacteria or viruses.

Although some have claimed that marijuana is an aphrodisiac, its validity as such is questionable. But the effects on the reproductive system is now certain. Marijuana diminishes both male and female reproductive hormones, which can cause a reduction in fertility by lowering sperm count and disrupting ovulation and the menstrual cycle. Marijuana is attached to high fat-containing areas in the body. The brain is one. So are ovaries and testicles.

10. Does marijuana use lead to other kinds of drug abuse?

Marijuana doesn't *automatically* lead to the use of heroin, cocaine, or other drugs, but it is a very important risk factor. In fact, nearly everyone who uses these other illicit drugs started with marijuana. That's why marijuana is referred to as a "gateway drug."

11. Is marijuana addicting?

Marijuana is an addicting drug—not in every case, but often enough for it to be a serious concern for anyone who uses it. *Addictive use* is defined by compulsive, repeated use in spite of adverse consequences. Marijuana's effects include tolerance, leading to dependence, and then inability to cease use. These properties are no different from any other drug whose patterns of use produce addictive disease.

Perhaps one reason so few people think marijuana isn't addicting is the confusion caused by the variety of state laws regarding marijuana. Many people think that because marijuana has been "decriminalized," it can't really be dangerous. Marijuana use and sale is still illegal in every state. Decriminalization means only that penalties have been reduced so that casual users do not get a criminal record.

12. How does marijuana affect teenagers?

Marijuana's greatest danger is its influence on the young. Because their bodies are still developing, the harmful effects of marijuana use can have long-range consequences. The psychological effects of the drug affect school performance, emotional and social development, and the users' set of values, all at a time when significant decisions about his or her life must be made. These effects can shape the child's entire life. For example, a teenager who uses marijuana to avoid anxiety about intimacy or personal interaction fails to develop important life skills.

The physical effects on the young are just as bad. As young people go through puberty, a healthy balance of male and female hormones is essential to normal maturation. Marijuana disrupts this process in adolescents just as it affects the reproductive systems of adults.

Young boys must have a normal amount of testosterone—a male hormone—during adolescence to transform their bones, bodies, facial hair, genitals, and voices to those of men. Marijuana seems to decrease this hormone in teenage boys. However, it increases testosterone in young girls, which can affect the normal functioning of the menstrual cycle and can provoke skin problems.

Also, of course, teenagers are more prone to traffic accidents, and marijuana contributes greatly to this trend. It is also bad for learning—the worst drug imaginable for someone who is going to school.

13. Does marijuana make you stupid?

Marijuana doesn't necessarily make you stupid— but it can make you *seem* stupid. Many scientists use the term *amotivational syndrome* to describe the effects that marijuana has on school and job performance. It means that marijuana users often don't seem to care much about learning or doing a good job; they're simply content to sit and watch life pass them by. Most teenagers who become heavily involved in drug use, for example, narrow their circle of friends and non-drug-related activities—in effect, shutting down whole areas of their lives. Whether physiologically or socially, it is clear that marijuana interferes with the brain's learning processes.

Fortunately, these effects are reversible. People who are treated for marijuana addiction can go on to live full, happy, and productive lives.

How to Manage Drug Use by Pregnant Women
Options for Prenatal Education, Counseling, and Referral

Establish Credibility and Show Concern

Women who are isolated from the primary culture by virtue of their poverty and ethnicity place a high value on personal contacts—they are most likely to believe information given by people they know and to follow the advice of those they trust and respect. They tend to be unconvinced by media campaigns, especially if they or their friends have had healthy babies and successful deliveries despite drug use.

Many low-income women are more concerned

The following plan for management of drug abuse among pregnant women was prepared by the American Council on Drug Education, and appeared in *Drugs and Pregnancy: It's Not Worth the Risk.* Copyright 1986, American Council for Drug Education. Used by permission; all rights reserved.

about the immediate pressures of day-to-day living than about future planning. For them, pregnancy is a natural state requiring little change or preventive care unless a real emergency occurs.

Family and friends are the dominant influences on these women's lives and powerful sources of information. Mothers and grandmothers especially are eager to give advice about prenatal care and are listened to willingly.

This close involvement with family often contrasts with their experience with the health care system. Many women express general dissatisfaction and frustration with the system—feeling doctors are too busy or important to explain what is happening and believing staff look down on them or are indifferent to their needs. Many minority women are also afraid to ask questions of their care givers.

Before any counseling or educational efforts will be accepted by the high risk pregnant woman, it is crucial to deal with her complaints and to establish the clinic as an alternative information source to her family. The best antidote to hazardous drug use during pregnancy is a strong therapeutic alliance between patient and practitioner focused on delivering a healthy baby and based on a genuine mutual respect.

Provide Personal Advice and Motivation for Each Patient

After a drug history has been completed and summarized, the primary practitioner should comment about the findings, conveying some basic facts to the patient about the potential hazards of continuing drug use during pregnancy. This individual attention should be given to every patient, whether or not she acknowledges any drug use in the history. It should only take a few moments of the first interview.

At this time, the drug habits of each woman should be reviewed and her risk classification validated. Those who are low risks—abstainers or only occasional users of legal drugs—usually need only one brief session with the primary physician followed by repeated reminders at subsequent prenatal visits, to avoid drug use. Those in a medium risk category generally benefit from additional group education. Most patients who are high risks for continued drug involvement need a regular schedule of individual counseling.*

In this brief but very personal meeting with the primary practitioner, each patient should be told:

1. We are here to help you have the healthiest baby possible. Each time you visit, we will be asking about some important health practices—such as your diet, drug use and exercise—and how we can help.
2. No one can guarantee an easy pregnancy and a healthy baby because many factors influence what happens. Some of these cannot be

---

* A referral for a substance abuse treatment evaluation is indicated, however, for those who do not respond to this individual attention within their normal prenatal services or for patients whose levels of use exceed those found in the "High" category. Immediate attention should be given to any patient using nontherapeutic doses of sedatives or tranquilizers or combining the use of barbiturates with alcohol.

changed, like your age, general health, family background, or weight when you got pregnant. BUT—there are some very important things you can do to reduce the risks. STOP SMOKING, DRINKING AND OTHER DRUG USE DURING PREGNANCY AND WHILE NURSING!

(The patient's personal risks and assets can be summarized here.) (See Figures 4 and 5.)

3. Even small risks can add up, and some are especially dangerous.
4. Cigarettes, alcohol, marijuana, and some medications may have either small or serious effects on childbearing. These effects depend on:
   • which drugs are used or mixed together;
   • the amounts taken;
   • how often drugs are used;
   • at what point in your baby's growth they are taken; and
   • you and your baby's sensitivities to the different drugs.

The worst effects follow the most use but even small effects are undesirable.

5. These drugs have been associated with miscarriages (spontaneous abortions) and stillbirths; complications of pregnancy and delivery like more bleeding; newborns who weigh too little to stay with their mothers safely because they were either born too soon or didn't grow enough in the womb; deformities of the baby's organs, arms, legs or face; irritable and restless infants who cry a lot and are difficult to feed; and children who remain small for their age, have behavior problems at home and

Have you taken any of these medications in the last six months?

MEDICATIONS	Check (✓) if yes	What brand (trademark) do you use?	When did you last use?	How much do you usually take?	How often do you usually use this?	Comments on: —How long use has continued —Reasons for use
1. PAIN KILLERS *ASPIRIN TYPE (acetylsalicylic acid) *TYLENOL TYPE (acetaminophen)						
2. COLD OR COUGH MEDICINES						
3. ALLERGY MEDICATIONS						
4. BIRTH CONTROL PILLS						
5. ACNE MEDICINES						
6. VITAMINS						
7. NAUSEA MEDICINES (morning sickness)						
8. ANTACIDS						
9. LAXATIVES						
10. ANTI-SEIZURE MEDICATIONS						
11. OTHER PRESCRIPTIONS						

FIGURE 4. Current medications.

238 APPENDIX B

Have you ever tried . . . . . . ?

DRUGS	Check (✓) if yes	How old were you when you first used?	When did you most recently use? If you quit, why?	How much do you usually use now?	Do you ever use more? How much?	How often do you usually use now?	Have you ever had problems from use?	Do you plan to quit now? How?	Comments on: —Reasons for use —Method of use/supply —Brand name
CIGARETTES									
ALCOHOL									
*BEER									
*WINE									
*LIQUOR									
MARIJUANA (pot, grass, reefer)									
STIMULANTS									
*DIET PILLS									
*AMPHETAMINES (speed)									
*COCAINE									
TRANQUILIZERS (Valium, Librium)									
SEDATIVES									
*SLEEPING PILLS									
*DOWNERS									
HALLUCINOGENS (LSD, PCP)									
INHALANTS (glue)									
OPIATES									
*HEROIN									
*METHADONE									

*Do you ever take any of these drugs together? If so, which ones and how often?

FIGURE 5. Drug use history.

school, and are retarded or don't do very well in school.

6. It's important for you to stop using these drugs while you are pregnant and to ask questions about possible dangers before you take any medications, including those you can buy in a drug store. Certainly, you should be VERY CAUTIOUS if you decide to use any drugs. Risks are lower when you use less. Avoid the use of anything that has not been specifically prescribed during pregnancy. Regular use of even small amounts of alcohol—as little as one drink a day—may cause your baby to weigh less. Avoid getting drunk or high with any drug while pregnant or nursing—the baby can also get dangerously "high." Especially avoid drug use in early pregnancy or during the last months before delivery.

The primary practitioner can reinforce this reminder about drug use with a simple but attractive and colorful pamphlet for the expectant mother to take home with her. If she is scheduled for a prenatal education class or individual counseling, the dates should be noted on an appointment card. Any additional services should coincide with her regular prenatal visits.

At each subsequent visit, the nurse or primary practitioner should inquire about any drug use during the intervening period. Congratulations are in order for any positive efforts that have been made. This regular monitoring can motivate the mother to keep trying if the benefits of abstinence are stressed and any gains are reinforced. Questions about drug use should be integrated with other questions about diet, water retention, weight gain, and so forth.

Offer Prenatal Education about Abusable Drugs

Women classified as medium drug risks need more motivation to quit and more assistance in planning how to stop. These can usually be provided most conveniently in a group. Groups can be regularly scheduled during clinic hours and conducted by staff assistants or trained volunteers. Counseling personnel from local substance abuse programs can provide useful suggestions about the structure and content of such groups and may be willing to train your staff or selected volunteers in how best to conduct one. Pregnant women referred to such groups should have their regular prenatal visits scheduled just before or after the group meeting.

Women should be invited to bring along their mothers, partners (spouses), or a trusted friend who will encourage them to have a healthier pregnancy. Research has shown that pregnant women are more likely to stop smoking and other drug use, eat an adequate diet, and follow other recommendations if they are encouraged by family members. All lifestyle changes should be understood and supported by their most influential relationships.

Prenatal groups will be more popular with most women and better attended if subjects other than drug use, such as comfort, appearance, physical/sexual activity and social or emotional problems are also emphasized. Each group should last at least an hour to allow time for questions and discussion. Because many low income or minority women are reluctant about participating in groups and revealing intimate details of their lives, discussion may be limited. If this happens, the group leader should bring up the subject and make sure the facts are given.

Three aspects of drug use should be examined:

1. Facts about the possible consequences of drug use during pregnancy should be discussed in detail with a special emphasis on risk levels. One objective should be to convince patients that the baby and not just themselves shares in the consequences of continued use.

2. Reasons why drugs are used should be discussed so potential strategies for quitting can be determined. It's important to know if a woman uses because her friends or partner use, because she's depressed or wants to escape.

3. Plans for quitting need to be made that recognize the real physical and emotional difficulties involved in changing habits, while at the same time, encouraging success in achieving a healthy lifestyle. Each woman should develop her own reasonable, practical and acceptable plan for discontinuing the drugs she is using—substituting alternative activities, making "contracts" with herself or others that detail rewards and punishments for specified actions, joining a self-help group, keeping a diary of the circumstances in which she is tempted, or whatever else makes sense. The PLAN, however, should be short term—lasting only until the next prenatal visit,

at which time it can be discussed and renewed or modified as necessary. Remember that these women often have a crisis orientation—immediate needs take precedence. The assistance of the father or a close family member/friend should be part of this plan, if at all possible.

The person who conducts this prenatal group can use audio-visual materials to reinforce the messages. These should match the understanding of the group members and their cultural or economic perspective—not suggesting, for example, that low-income women go on a vacation or hire a babysitter to "get away for awhile" if they are depressed or overwhelmed by other responsibilities. Realistic solutions need to be offered.

The group leader should be hopeful as well as concerned. She should stress the mother's very real ability to reduce the risks of an unhealthy baby and to care for her infant. Threats of dire outcomes and tales of horrible "monsters" should *not* be used. Neither should the clinic staff reprimand the pregnant woman about "slips" or make predictions about any terrible consequences from intoxication. These comments are likely to backfire.

Counsel High-Risk Users Individually

Pregnant women who are heavy drug users require individual attention. They may attend a group education class but they also need a complete diagnostic evaluation by an experienced substance abuse treatment professional to validate their drug-use history and assess their strengths and coping skills. Hospital-affiliated clinics may have social workers or psychologists who can do this.[1,2]

Once a plan for abstinence or a monitored reduction in use, or transfer to an approved drug regimen (e.g., methadone maintenance) is developed that is acceptable to the expectant mother, individual counseling may be conducted by staff from the regular prenatal service. It is better to have patients supervised in one place, if at all possible, so that alliances with clinicians are strengthened. Much of the guidance that is required is practical rather than specialized. Half-hour sessions, scheduled from one to four times a month when the woman ordinarily comes to the clinic, are usually sufficient. A program for alcohol abusing pregnant women at Boston City Hospital found that two-thirds of the heavy drinkers who came to individual counseling sessions conducted by regular prenatal clinic staff stopped abusive drinking after two or three visits. Most reduced their drinking within two weeks.

The focus of individual sessions should be on the individual's real life situations and the circumstances that are associated with continued drug use. Is she having difficulties with her partner or does she feel abandoned by him? Is there an ambivalence about this pregnancy that needs to be resolved? Is she self-medicating serious depression with alcohol or other drugs? Does she need to find friends who can have fun without drugs and not pressure her to use? Any period of abstinence should be praised and the patient should be reassured that there are always benefits from quitting—even late in pregnancy. Usually, women who use drugs heavily and find them difficult to give up, even when the benefits to the developing baby are obvious, have very low self esteem and badly need support and reinforcement. They may be fearful of the birth process, upset by their changed appearance, or fearful of the financial problems related to having a child. These concerns need to be shared. The assistance of a family member can be a great asset.

Refer Drug Abusers Who Don't Respond

If a pregnant woman does not respond to individual counseling at the prenatal clinic within a few weeks and continues heavy drug use, or is too disruptive for staff to handle, a referral should be made to a specialized agency or facility. The choice will depend on the needs and circumstances of the woman and the availability of services in the community. Help in making a selection and a referral can usually be found through the State Substance Abuse Prevention and Treatment Agency or listings under alcohol or drug treatment in the local telephone book.

Arrangements should be explored with staff at the programs under consideration before a referral is completed. Make certain that costs can be covered, transportation is available, the woman is willing to enroll, her family will encourage her participation, and the services are really suitable. Patients may need services ranging from detoxification to group homes to a specialized outpatient clinic.

Usually, the primary practitioner continues to have basic responsibility for prenatal care and should coordinate these services until the baby is born. Many drug-abusing women can benefit from continued treatment for substance abuse and from counseling to improve their parenting skills after delivery.

Dr. Barry Zuckerman, an expert on the developmental consequences of maternal drug use, observes:

> Children of drug abusers may be subject to double jeopardy. They may suffer in utero effects on their central nervous system associated with drug abuse and then suffer from poor environmental circumstances due to nonoptimal parenting associated with a drug user's lifestyle.[3]

By intervening at the earliest stages in pregnancy, the caregiver takes advantage of a rare opportunity to interrupt a cruel and doubly destructive behavioral pattern. The fact is that drug abuse is deleterious to both childbearing and childrearing. When a drug problem is identified and addressed, not only does the pregnant woman's physical condition improve, but her mental and emotional capacity for motherhood is enhanced immensely. In the long term, this may be the most enduring and most significant outcome of the physician's involvement.

References

1. Finnegan LP (ed): Drug Dependence in Pregnancy: Clinical Management of Mother and Child. NIDA Research Monograph. Rockville, MD, Department of Health and Human Services, 1979.
2. Rosett HL, Weiner L: *Alcohol and the Fetus: A Clinical Perspective.* New York, Oxford University Press, 1984.
3. Pinkert TM (ed): Current Research on the Consequences of Maternal Drug Abuse. NIDA Research Monograph 59. Rockville, MD, Department of Health and Human Services, 1979.

Index

Developmental history, in
dependency diagnosis,
107–109, 120–122, 135–
137, 153–156, 165–168
*Diagnostic and Statistical Manual
of Mental Disorders-III*, 97
Disease concept, of
dependency, 190–191
Dissociation of ideas, 43–44, 86
Dopamine, 48
Driving performance, 44–46
Drug abuse. *See* Substance
abuse
Drug abuse prevention. *See*
Prevention, of drug
abuse

Education
for drug abuse prevention,
204, 217–218
as prenatal drug abuse
program component,
234, 239, 240–242
Emphysema, 62
Endocrine system, marijuana
effects, 226
Enzyme immunoassay, for
marijuana detection, 176,
177, 180–181, 182
Estrogen, 71
Euphoria, 86
Europe
as marijuana supply source,
10
marijuana use in, 8

Family
attitude towards drugs, 207

Family (*Cont.*)
marijuana abuse prevention
efforts, 206–212
marijuana addiction
treatment involvement,
196–198
prenatal drug abuse
management
involvement, 234, 240
Family dynamics, in
dependency diagnosis,
109–110, 122–123, 137–
138
Family psychiatric history, 107,
120, 134, 153, 164–165
Family therapy, 195
Fertility, marijuana and, 70, 71,
226–227
Fetal alcohol syndrome, 72
Fetal growth retardation, 71–72
Follicle-stimulating hormone,
69–70

Ganja, 6. *See also* Marijuana
Gateway concept, of substance
abuse, 25–28, 227
Genetic factors, in dependency,
101
Gonadotropin, 70, 71
Grass, 6. *See also* Marijuana
Group therapy, 195

Hallucinations, 44, 86
Hallucinogens, 12–14
Hashish
definition, 223–224
potency, 6
preparation, 6

252